'Many women who have experienced sexual abuse find giving birth traumatising. Using vivid and moving case studies, this book offers excellent guidance on supporting those women to have a better experience of pregnancy, labour and birth. It will be an invaluable resource for health professionals working in this area.'

– *Kim Thomas, CEO, Birth Trauma Association*

'Kicki's book is a compelling reminder that being treated with kindness, dignity and respect is the number one source of safety in maternity care. Practical, accessible and with the voices of survivors threaded through every page, this is a must-read for all those who aspire to trauma-informed and human-rights-centred practice.'

– *Maria Booker, Programmes Director, Birthrights*

'It is great to see a book dedicated to guiding health professionals to support survivors of sexual abuse when they are pregnant and giving birth. This is an area of maternity care that can cause exacerbation of trauma for women if handled poorly and the opportunity for growth and healing if handled well. The health provider sits in that juncture between further trauma and a pathway to healing and this is a serious responsibility that can weigh heavily on us without guidance. This book provides that guidance.'

– *Hannah Dahlen, Professor of Midwifery,*
Western Sydney University

'This book is so needed – although I truly wish it wasn't. We need more empathy in the birth room, so that no woman needs to feel she has to disclose her history in order to be treated with gentleness and respect.'

– *Milli Hill, Founder of the Positive Birth Movement and author of*
The Positive Birth Book *and* Give Birth Like a Feminist

T0271471

'This is a very important area to address, and the content will be very useful for the target audience. The integration of women's stories provides very effective insights into what matters for pregnant women who have experienced sexual abuse specifically, and for pregnant women in general.'

– Soo Downe, Professor of Midwifery Studies, UCLan

Supporting Survivors of Sexual Abuse Through Pregnancy and Childbirth

of related interest

The Business of Maternity Care
A Guide for Midwives and Doulas Setting Up in Private Practice
Denise Tiran
ISBN 978 1 84819 386 4
eISBN 978 0 85701 385 9

Complementary Therapies in Maternity Care
An Evidence-Based Approach
Denise Tiran
ISBN 978 1 84819 328 4
eISBN 978 0 85701 284 5

Aromatherapy in Midwifery Practice
Denise Tiran
ISBN 9781 84819 288 1
eISBN 978 0 85701 235 7

Choices in Pregnancy and Childbirth
A Guide to Options for Health Professionals, Midwives,
Holistic Practitioners, and Parents
John Wilks
ISBN 978 1 84819 219 5
eISBN 978 0 85701 167 1

Supporting Survivors of Sexual Abuse Through Pregnancy and Childbirth

A Guide for Midwives, Doulas and Other Healthcare Professionals

KICKI HANSARD

Forewords by Penny Simkin and
Phyllis Klaus

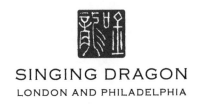

SINGING DRAGON
LONDON AND PHILADELPHIA

Extracts from Simkin and Klaus (2004) throughout the book are reproduced
with kind permission from Penny Simkin and Phyllis Klaus.

First published in 2020
by Singing Dragon
an imprint of Jessica Kingsley Publishers
73 Collier Street
London N1 9BE, UK
and
400 Market Street, Suite 400
Philadelphia, PA 19106, USA

www.singingdragon.com

Copyright © Kicki Hansard 2020
Foreword copyright © Penny Simkin 2020
Foreword copyright © Phyllis Klaus 2020

All rights reserved. No part of this publication may be reproduced in any
material form (including photocopying, storing in any medium by electronic
means or transmitting) without the written permission of the copyright owner
except in accordance with the provisions of the law or under terms of a licence
issued in the UK by the Copyright Licensing Agency Ltd. www.cla.co.uk or in
overseas territories by the relevant reproduction rights organisation, for details
see www.ifrro.org. Applications for the copyright owner's written permission to
reproduce any part of this publication should be addressed to the publisher.

Warning: The doing of an unauthorised act in relation to a copyright work
may result in both a civil claim for damages and criminal prosecution.

Library of Congress Cataloging in Publication Data
A CIP catalog record for this book is available from the Library of Congress

British Library Cataloguing in Publication Data
A CIP catalogue record for this book is available from the British Library

ISBN 978 1 84819 424 3
eISBN 978 0 85701 377 4

Printed and bound in Great Britain

Disclaimer

The author of this book does not dispense medical advice or prescribe the use of any technique as a form of treatment for physical or medical problems without the advice of a physician, either directly or indirectly. The intent of the author is only to offer information of a general nature to help you in your quest for emotional and spiritual wellbeing. In the event you use any of the information in this book for yourself, the author and the publisher assume no responsibility for your actions.

Contents

Contents

Foreword

Kicki Hansard honoured me when she asked me to write a foreword to this book. As a leader in maternity care in the UK and beyond, she has chosen to devote much time and energy to improving the maternity experiences of sexual abuse survivors, by explaining to maternity care providers the unique needs of sexual abuse survivors as they experience pregnancy, childbirth and parenthood.

The book opens with a powerful and enlightening, though very disturbing, poem – 'I didn't expect you to know, but...' – by a survivor, 'Melanie', in which she addresses her maternity caregivers. In verse after verse, Melanie describes various incidents in her labour and birth care that caused pain, shame, violation, sense of failure, weakness, inability to speak for herself and even physical assault. Then the poem shifts its focus to 'What if...care was' sensitive, individualised, trauma-informed, compassionate, free from ego and the need to protect women from themselves? The poem progresses, showing us how, over several subsequent births, her hurt was transformed to anger, and finally, in the last stanza 'Empowered, informed and healed', Melanie is 'no longer a victim'. A poignant account of Post-traumatic Growth.

Sexual abuse is particularly damaging (often unexpectedly so) to survivors when they become pregnant. The same parts of the body are affected by both. While pregnancy is often considered a joyous and wanted experience, sexual abuse is absolutely the opposite.

Many women and their caregivers are unaware of the profound negative effects that can result from early abuse. Their lack of understanding often results in care that is thoughtless and that triggers memories of abuse. Women often come away from birth, not only with their baby, but also with a feeling that they were helpless and inadequate – abused yet again.

With this book, which primarily addresses maternity caregivers, Kicki Hansard offers insight on the many ways childbirth is perceived by sexual abuse survivors. To give life to her narrative, she includes the heart-felt graphic descriptions of the experiences of dozens of survivors whom she surveyed for the book. Kicki also draws heavily from the literature on the topic and her own observations as a doula and childbirth educator, working with survivors.

This narrative is a compelling portrayal of the challenges facing sexual abuse survivors. The net effect on the reader may well be a mix of guilt ('How could I have done that?') and understanding ('That explains why she tensed up and cried when I did vaginal exams!'; 'I can see why she couldn't trust me!').

Kicki offers much information on the impact of sexual abuse on the individual and through each phase of childbearing, providing advice and suggestions for caregivers on the importance of listening carefully and compassionately, and making informed decision-making and human rights the centre of good care. This topic is especially complicated for caregivers who may believe that some choices of the parents may be dangerous for the baby or mother. Of course, this issue is not easily dealt with in any branch of medicine. Kicki deals with this controversial topic in Chapter 3, along with such heavy topics as vicarious traumatisation of the caregiver, improving communication between client and caregiver, issues around touching clients, and many other emotionally charged topics. The book includes inspiring examples of 'Healing Through Birth', stories from survivors for whom their birth experience resulted in what is often referred to as Post-traumatic Growth (becoming stronger than ever as a result of struggling with the effects of the abuse and overcoming them).

The book ends with birth stories, and 'Top Tips' for care providers from the women who participated in the survey are given throughout the book. These are worth reflection and discussion with colleagues.

This book will educate and inspire, but because it is also critical of much that occurs in maternity care, including Kicki's passionate advocacy and strong opinions, the book will provoke disagreement, resistance and self-doubt in readers. I hope they will evaluate their own perceptions of this topic, discuss it with colleagues, try the suggestions that Kicki offers for improving care of birthing survivors, and find they can embrace trauma-informed care to improve the maternity care experiences of sexual abuse survivors.

Penny Simkin, Physical Therapist, Educator, Author and Birth Counsellor
Senior Faculty, Simkin Center for Allied Birth Vocations
at Bastyr University, Kenmore, Washington, USA

Foreword

Kicki Hansard's book *Supporting Survivors of Sexual Abuse Through Pregnancy and Childbirth: A Guide for Midwives, Doulas and Other Healthcare Professionals* is a clarion call to all caregivers to become aware of the deleterious power of negative words, attitudes and actions on a birthing woman and most especially on a survivor of sexual abuse. The emotional pain of such behavioural mistreatment adds insult to injury to a woman survivor who already is holding bodily and emotional pain.

Hansard's sensitive questionnaire resulted in numerous personal responses from women survivors of sexual abuse. Her research has added to current knowledge of women's abuse experiences. Sensitive and aware caregivers will be saddened, appalled and disgusted that their fellow colleagues could be so unaware of the effects of their actions. Reading this book should be a catalyst to uninformed caregivers whose actions heretofore may have been extremely detrimental to the survivor. Hopefully, they will become enlightened by the information in this book.

Aside from women's descriptions, poignantly and painfully described, Hansard gives useful antidotes to those problems of birth with excellent methods for help and healing. All is not lost. All of us as caregivers, at times, need to look at the effect of what we think is right for a woman versus how she perceives it. My hope for all my fellow caregiving colleagues is to read this book, learn from it and move forward. It's important to read the whole book and you will be relieved to find new and creative ways to meet the challenges that survivors of abuse face in their maternity experience.

Phyllis Klaus, LMFT, LMSW, co-author of *When Survivors Give Birth: Understanding and Healing the Effects of Early Sexual Abuse on Childbearing Women, The Doula Book, Bonding,* and *Your Amazing Newborn*

About This Book

This book was written with support and stories from female survivors of sexual abuse and that is why throughout this book, I'm using the feminine pronoun. That is not to exclude anyone who identifies with another gender or no gender at all.

It might appear as though all the perpetrators mentioned are male but that is not to say that women do not perpetrate sexual abuse.

The book is written in the first person because I want you, the reader, to feel as if we are having a conversation about this topic rather than making it feel as though it has been written for a fictional third person.

The quotes are verbatim extracts from questionnaires that were completed by survivors who volunteered to help with this book for which I am eternally grateful.

I'm choosing to talk about the women in this book as survivors of abuse rather than victims as the use of that word feels so paralysing and implies helplessness and pity while someone who is a survivor adapts to their environment and is in control of their own destiny. I admire the strength and courage of women who are survivors of sexual abuse and violence.

Some of the names are the women's real names and some have been changed on the request of the women.

I didn't expect you to know...but

*Your rough vaginal examinations and failure to stop, even
as I cried, evoked those feelings of shame. Shame on me
for being too weak to stop this from happening to me.*

*When you told me to stop making a fuss, I
heard words that destroyed my soul.*

*When you told me I'd not be able to give birth, that
my body had failed me, you just compounded my
lack of faith in my body to do anything good.*

*Your patronising 'good girl' when I was compliant
and silent sent shivers through me.*

*I didn't expect you to know...but when you
did things to my body or simply*

told me you were going to do them, you violated me all over again.

*When you all left me naked on the operating table,
you exposed my deep-rooted vulnerability.*

*When you spoke about me, not to me even though I was there, you
took away my power again. Your failure to acknowledge me was just
hushed conversations with the decisions being made for me yet again.*

*When you grabbed my breast from the mouth of my baby,
squeezed it into a shape and rammed it back into her mouth, my
already loathing of my breasts became unbearable. Your actions
ensured I'd fail to breastfeed four out of five of my babies.*

*I didn't expect you to know but should I have needed to tell you
that I was sexually abused by my stepfather during my childhood?*

*The way you treated me during pregnancy and birth
triggered memories of his words and actions, you
opened a path for his wickedness to enter my space, the
one place I wanted unmarred by his presence.*

So, here's a what if...

What if care for ALL women could be based on an assumption that everything could be triggering to anyone in obstetrics and gynaecology care?

What if kind, compassionate and emotionally sensitive care was for everyone, given by everyone?

What if egos and the need to save women from themselves were left outside of the birthing spaces?

Maybe, just maybe the change would be profound!

You see, your 'silly girl' comment that was made during my last pregnancy with my fifth baby about me making choices surrounding my birth, no longer hurt me but made me angry.

Empowered, informed and healed, I am a woman, an intelligent autonomous woman.

Most of all I am no longer a victim.

Melanie – survivor

Introduction

The effect of childhood sexual abuse and sexual violence does not end when the abuse ends or when the assault is over; instead they continue to cause havoc and upset and the impact is often deep and long lasting. When a survivor of childhood sexual abuse reaches childbearing age and becomes pregnant, many issues related to the abuse can re-surface, often quite unexpectedly, as pregnancy, childbirth and breastfeeding can present challenges for a survivor. Her body is changing as her belly is growing and, at some point, she will start to feel the baby moving inside her. Her breasts are swelling and growing in size and they can often feel tender. For the woman who is a survivor of sexual violence, it might feel like she's losing autonomy and control of her body and any interaction with caregivers where she doesn't feel heard could remind her of the assailant in the past who ignored her pleas to stop.

During the time when a woman is pregnant, she will usually be meeting with health professionals more often than she might have ever done in her whole life previously. During these meetings with a doctor or midwife, she will often be asked questions about her diet and personal life and measurements and samples are taken from her body. This can evoke memories and make women feel like they have lost all control of their body again and can make them feel uncomfortable, even at times quite disturbed to be subjected to these inspections on a regular basis. As the focus may appear to be, and often is, all on the baby, while the woman is being told to eat a certain way and to do regular exercise for the sake of the baby, this might feel humiliating to her, especially if she's been neglected and made to feel like she was less important than someone else in her past.

A rape victim might find herself giving birth to her baby back in the same hospital where she was examined and evidence collected after her attack. She might be trying to tell the staff that she's in pain and scared but they might not be listening to her, just like when the rape happened. She might start to howl and fight to get away from the situation or become quiet and compliant. Her behaviour might leave care providers feeling confused and perplexed, assuming that this is the way this woman handles labour and birth. Some might show empathy and kindness; others might get angry and try to take control of the situation.

There are some amazing, caring and dedicated health professionals out there, supporting and caring for women in maternity services. However, many care providers are unaware of the impact that sexual abuse has on the women that they look after. The woman who is a survivor will often be labelled as difficult and noncompliant even though all that she is doing and the way she is behaving is to protect herself because she might be feeling exactly the way she felt when she was abused. She might even find herself having flashbacks to the traumatic event. Survivors often don't know how to deal with the feelings that re-surface and it could be the case that a survivor cannot even recall the abuse, especially if it happened during childhood; if so, this will feel very confusing.

I believe that if care providers had a way of recognising and acknowledging the needs that these women present, they would be able to adapt their care accordingly. All that might be needed is something as simple as always knocking on the door before entering the room the woman is in or lowering the body to be on the same level as the woman when speaking to her and ensuring that the use of language is not demeaning or triggering.

So many light bulbs went on in my head when I first got my hands on the book *When Survivors Give Birth* written by Penny Simkin and Phyllis Klaus (2004). It all made so much sense! Of course, as a doula I had encountered women who found it difficult to agree to vaginal exams and feared needles used to collect blood or give injections. There were women I'd supported who were extremely worried about being naked or exposing their body and felt very suspicious of medical authority figures. There were women who would compile very detailed and lengthy birth plans, stating everything they didn't want (rather than what their wishes were) and whose labour often ended with the medical classification of 'failure to progress', often for no obvious reason. Many of these women also felt a profound disappointment with previous births and were upset, often angry, with many of the caregivers involved before and during their experience.

I had no idea that all these different behaviours could, in fact, be the result of childhood sexual abuse or sexual violence in these women's past: abuse that they might not have any memory of and might only be returning to them as they experience the intensity of labour and hear words and phrases that trigger memories buried deep down in their unconscious minds.

I believe every single care provider needs to take responsibility for how women are treated and cared for in maternity services as I'm sure no one would want to cause more trauma to someone who has already survived so much. The Hippocratic Oath states: 'First, do no harm' but unfortunately, I believe that, due to the lack of education, resources and staff, many medical healthcare providers re-traumatise survivors of abuse as well as causing long-term mental health issues for many women. There is even a word for it, 'iatrogenic', which relates to an adverse effect or complication resulting from medical treatment or advice. There are interventions and interference in the physiological birth process happening daily on the maternity wards across this country that leads to traumatisation as well as re-traumatisation. All are carried out in the name of good care.

Women often say to me that they had not considered that being a survivor of sexual abuse would have an impact on their pregnancy, birth and postnatal experience. That it had never occurred to them that what they had survived would come back and haunt them during what should be one of the happiest times in their life. They often feel anger at their perpetrators who did so much damage to them at the time and still have the power to continue to damage them and their relationships, not only with caregivers, but also with their partners and, sometimes, even their babies.

There are very few books specifically aimed at health professionals about supporting survivors during pregnancy, childbirth and the postnatal period. Often survivors are the women that get labelled as difficult, aggressive and unreasonable patients. These women might dissociate during labour and lash out when someone gets too near or triggers a survival response, buried in their body's cellular memory. I sometimes hear health professionals state that violence is never acceptable but if they could only understand that these women are fighting for their lives, they might be more forgiving and look at other approaches or ways to communicate so that they can support these women better. Whilst I do not condone how these women are reacting and always believe violence is unhelpful, I do think it is important and it makes a lot of sense to understand why these women might be reacting and behaving the way they do. Everyone is the way they are for a reason and, as care providers, we might become the target of violent reactions but our aim should always be to find a way to offer support that works.

In this book, I will start by defining sexual abuse and look at what we know about sexual abuse in Chapter 1. How widespread is it? What research is there about sexual abuse and how does it impact pregnancy, childbirth and the postnatal period? How does trauma influence the behaviour of a survivor? I will also take a look at the things that women need during labour and birth.

In Chapter 2, I will give information and support aimed at those of us who support survivors during pregnancy and childbirth. Are there some ways to identify survivors and how can we respond to survivors when they try to disclose their past to us? Should we even ask? We will look at triggers, what they are and how we must all be mindful to avoid routine procedures becoming more important than the women that we support. In this chapter, survivors also share what kind of support will be helpful and what support has the potential to re-traumatise.

Chapter 3 considers the legal issues surrounding consent and human rights in an obstetric setting. What impact might sexual violence have on the pregnant and labouring woman and her relationship with her body? Language really matters in maternity care and I will discuss alternative ways of gaining information and supporting in a respectful and caring way, at times signposting to other services, for example, mental health support. What are the top tips from survivors to care providers?

Chapter 4 deals with practical ideas for supporting survivors during the postnatal period and looks at infant feeding and perinatal mental health as well as ideas about how to support and help women move on from and process difficult birth experiences.

In Chapter 5, we will look at some positive stories to show how positive pregnancy, birth and postnatal experiences can form an important part of the process of healing from sexual violence and a way for the woman to re-claim her body.

In the final chapter, I will be summarising what has been covered and, I hope, making my voice heard in calling for work to be done to honour women, their rights and their choices during childbirth. Not just survivors of abuse but all women.

I'm not an expert on trauma or sexual violence (or an expert on anything in fact) and, as far as I know, I'm not a survivor of childhood sexual abuse or sexual violence. However, I have studied both sociology and psychology as part of my degree and I have worked as a doula and doula course facilitator since 2002 when I've had the opportunity to experience and see how women are cared for in labour and childbirth. I've worked with many survivors; some of them told me beforehand, others told me afterwards or even during the birth and some never told me but everything that I witnessed would have made total sense if they were survivors.

There have been times when I've felt so frustrated and even angry when, on rare occasions, I've seen some care providers treat women badly when, in my view, it usually doesn't take much effort to be kind, caring and respectful. It costs nothing, apart from an investment of time from the person in question, and it makes the biggest difference for all women, not just those who have been through abuse and violence, though it is especially important for those women. I'm glad to say that I see kind and compassionate care the majority of the time from health professionals who are doing an amazing job in a maternity health system that is in great need of more investment, more staff and other resources. The Royal College of Midwives (RCM) reported back in 2017 that the NHS maternity service was 'reaching crisis point', with England alone short of 3500 midwives (RCM 2017).

What care providers, doctors, midwives, doulas, sonographers, paediatricians, maternity care assistants, health visitors, receptionists and everyone who comes into contact with a pregnant woman must remember is that the way we treat a woman during labour, birth and postnatally will stay with that woman forever. If your treatment of her triggers memories of previous abuse and traumatises that woman, she could potentially remember you as a perpetrator. It's time for us all to ask ourselves: how do I want to be remembered?

This book is written with a heavy influence from Simkin and Klaus's book *When Survivors Give Birth* (2004), my bible and go-to book to ensure that I'm always providing compassionate and dignified care not just for survivors of abuse but for all women. If you are a maternity care worker, you must add this book to your library. It will completely open your eyes to the damage you might be doing, unknowingly, on a daily basis.

My hope is that by writing this book, short, concise and to the point, I can help everyone who comes into contact with a woman during pregnancy, childbirth and in the postnatal period to feel better equipped with some tools that they can use to adapt the care they provide. I also hope to kindle a willingness to take into account the impact they will have on this woman's memory of her birth experience.

I'm extremely grateful to the women who shared with me their experiences of their own treatment in maternity care as survivors of abuse and sexual violence as well as the many clients I've worked with, who have all shown me how much of a difference the little things made to their healing and recovery. Women will always be my greatest teachers and I feel honoured and grateful for learning so much from each and every one of them.

Chapter 1

What We Know

The definition and prevalence of sexual abuse

The definition of sexual violence taken from the Centre for Action on Rape and Abuse website (2016) states:

> Sexual violence is any unwanted sexual act or activity. It includes rape, sexual assault, child sexual abuse (CSA), sexual harassment, female genital mutilation, trafficking, sexual exploitation, and ritual abuse.

Simkin and Klaus talk about different types of CSA in their book *When Survivors Give Birth* (2004) and they classify the abuse into three different activities which cause sexual arousal in the abuser or in someone else.

- Physical abuse: rape as in being forced to have vaginal, anal or oral sex; being touched without consent, for example, pinching, patting, embracing, rubbing, groping, flicking, kissing and fondling, being touched on the breasts, bottom, legs, etc. In some abusive relationships, physical abuse can be followed by favouritism and flattery.
- Psychological abuse: exposing the genitals to a child, voyeurism, intrusive interest in the sexual development of the child, exposure to pornographic content or other inappropriate sexual behaviour.
- Verbal abuse: erotic talk or innuendo, accusations of 'sexy', 'loose', 'whore-like' behaviour or explicit language.

We will probably never know the exact numbers of sexual abuse and assault as many survivors are shackled by shame and fearful of the consequences of speaking out. Recent campaigns such as the #metoo social media explosion seemed to suggest that there are very few women who have never been subjected to some form of sexual harassment.

Figures from the Crime Survey for England and Wales (Office for National Statistics 2017), show that 1 in 5 women have experienced some form of sexual violence since the age of 16. The NSPCC reports that 31 per cent of young women aged 18–24 report having experienced sexual abuse in childhood (Radford *et al.* 2011). Other studies show that 1 in 3 teenage girls in England have been pressured into doing something sexual by a partner (Wood *et al.* 2015) and a third of female students in the UK have experienced inappropriate touching or groping at university (*The Telegraph* 2015).

These statistics paint a somewhat painful picture of the prevalence of sexual abuse in our society and mean that most birth workers will almost definitely at some point be supporting women during the childbearing years who are survivors of some form of sexual violence although many will never disclose this to them or perhaps even to anyone.

We might not have an exact percentage figure of how many women have experienced sexual abuse, in childhood as well as in adulthood. However, what we do know is that these women are at risk of re-traumatisation during childbearing as many of the processes and procedures carried out by the woman's caregivers during pregnancy and childbirth potentially imitate situations from the abuse that could trigger memories and strong emotions in survivors (Garratt 2010).

Studies show us that 94 per cent of women who have been raped develop Post-traumatic Stress Disorder (PTSD) so we have to consider survivors as being traumatised and needing some help and support with healing from the trauma (Riggs, Murdock and Walsh 1992).

We know that the traumatic experience of sexual abuse and violence, whenever in a woman's life it took place, has a powerful effect on the survivor and influences their worldview, health and behaviour. We all experience and interpret events and situations we find ourselves in individually so the easiest thing to do, as birth workers, is to adapt a trauma-informed approach with every woman that we work with. I truly believe that in the future it will be compulsory to educate everyone who works with people in any setting in trauma-informed care.

Trauma-informed care is a way of addressing the consequences of trauma and supporting healing and is not a form of treatment or intervention but rather a way of being. The core principles of trauma-informed care centre around:

- Safety – creating a space where women feel culturally, emotionally and physically safe as well as having an awareness of each individual's discomfort or unease.
- Transparency and trustworthiness – providing full and accurate information about what's happening and what's likely to happen next.
- Choice – the recognition of the need for an approach that honours an individual's dignity.
- Collaboration and mutuality – this is achieved through the recognition that healing happens in relationships and partnerships with shared decision-making.
- Empowerment – given by the recognition of an individual's strengths. These strengths are built on and validated.

Dignified, kind and empathetic maternity care should be at the top of every hospital's agenda.

The impact of sexual abuse

In her book, *Trauma and Recovery: The Aftermath of Violence – From Domestic Abuse to Political Terror,* Judith Herman (1997) draws parallels between the experiences of survivors of rape and childhood sexual abuse and the experiences of survivors of war. She concludes that the same psychological syndrome, PTSD, is affecting both groups and that the fear and panic the survivors experienced in their past will continue to influence their lives in the future.

Many survivors of sexual abuse blame their body as the abuse usually takes place on a physical level. They might also have felt bodily sensations associated with the abuse which bring shame and disgust. Survivors might see their body as an inconvenience or annoyance as, at the time when it should have resisted an attack, it surrendered and by doing that, in a sense, it let them down. Some survivors even view their body as dysfunctional and broken because of what happened to them.

As a way of avoiding being aware of the feeling in their bodies during the abuse, many survivors learn how to avoid paying close and careful attention to what their body is communicating to them, not only about what is going on inside them but also what the body might need. This might mean not emptying the bladder when the urge comes, instead holding the urine in until they choose to go, or other survivors might push themselves to extremes in terms of food and exercise. Survivors might even cause harm to their bodies and are often at an increased risk of developing an addiction (Courtois 1996). This can be viewed as a form of coping strategy or avoidance defence to be able to handle the pain, humiliation and fear of the abuse. It's not unusual for survivors to carry this with them for the rest of their lives, with it eventually becoming part of their persona. It forms part of the great need many survivors have to be in control of as much as they can in their lives.

The trauma of sexual abuse also affects the neurological and hormonal systems in the body as well as the immune system. We know that the emotional state of a person will have an impact on their physical wellbeing. Studies show that survivors of sexual abuse report more somatic symptoms and discomfort compared to people who are not survivors, as well as a greater degree of chronic disease (Lang *et al.* 2010). The most common and most general are: gastrological diseases, stomach diseases (e.g. ulcers), respiratory disorders (e.g. asthma, bronchitis, emphysema), heart problems, hypertension, arthritis, diabetes and gynaecological problems. Gynaecological problems are most often related to the loss of the menstrual cycle or excessive bleeding, sexual dysfunctions, frequent pains in the lower abdomen (even when not during menstruation), frequent inflammation of genitalia and pains during sexual intercourse (Rodgers *et al.* 2003).

A study looked at the association between fibromyalgia syndrome and previous emotional, physical and sexual abuse and found a link; however, more robust studies are needed (Häuser *et al.* 2011).

When it comes to medical examination of someone who has been through trauma it is often impossible to find the source or reasons for many of the symptoms that a survivor might be expressing. The person might be experiencing physical pain; however, no physical injuries can be found which can often mean that the pain is psychosomatic, that is, stemming from a psychological disorder, such as stress. Any traumatic event usually has an impact on the structure and function of the brain as well as on the health of the physical body and a person's psyche.

Scaer (2005) noticed that in some cases, trauma could lead to serious psychiatric disorders, depending on the severity of the trauma. He also believed that a number of the physical complaints he saw in his patients were caused by a specific experience in that patient's life and not by any damage to individual organs.

Other general health issues as a result of sexual abuse are the risk of exposure to infections or sexually transmitted diseases (STDs). There is also the increased risk that the survivor will get involved in abusive relationships in the future. There are some studies that highlight the fact that a person who has been raped will be more likely to be subjected to physical violence in a relationship when compared to someone who has not been raped (e.g. Brener *et al.* 1999).

It can be difficult for a sexually abused child to relax as it often feels safer to be vigilant and ready, in case something bad is about to happen. Many of the psychosomatic problems associated with sexual abuse are caused by the persistent stimulation of the autonomic nervous system, which is releasing the stress hormones epinephrine and cortisol and this has a long-term health impact on the body. This often results in a weakened immune system, leaving survivors more likely to catch colds and suffering from chronic fatigue and exhaustion.

It is worth noting that for some survivors every bodily change or sensation dominates their minds to the exclusion of everything else. Even the slightest sign of illness could put them into an uncontrollable spin of panic and discomfort.

I believe this to be relevant and important information when it comes to understanding how sexual abuse impacts women during pregnancy and childbirth.

How trauma influences behaviour

There is quite a selection of different research out there about the impact of childhood sexual abuse on childbearing women (see the References section). We know that research into the area of post-traumatic stress shows that the body continues to behave as if it is being traumatised even if the actual traumatic event occurred many years ago (Iribarren *et al.* 2005). If a traumatising experience is re-triggered by reminders of that trauma, the body will react with a conditioned response. In other words, it happens on a subconscious level which means it can even come as a surprise for the person who is being triggered.

The human brain with its unique properties has evolved over thousands of generations and is capable of absorbing and storing more information than that of any other species on our planet. The lower parts of the brain are receiving information from the outside world through our five senses: smell, sight, taste, sound and touch. There is also information gathered in the body, telling us where we are in space, how much oxygen we have, things about our heart, muscles and lungs which are also sent as signals to the lower parts of the brain. All this information is continuously monitored, stored and acted on throughout the day. This helps us keep our system in equilibrium, to keep us healthy, safe and, fundamentally, alive.

The lower parts of the brain are simpler and more reactive and the further up the brain we move, the more complex the brain becomes. The top level, the neo-cortex, handles the most complex human functions such as interpreting touch, vision and hearing, as well as speech, reasoning, emotions, learning and fine control of movement. Right below this region is the limbic area, which controls emotional content and responses. Further down, we have the cerebellum, which is in charge of co-ordinating muscle movements, maintaining posture, and balance. Lastly, the lowest part of the brain performs many of the automatic functions such as breathing, heart rate, body temperature, wake and sleep cycles, digestion, sneezing, coughing, vomiting, swallowing and, guess what, childbirth.

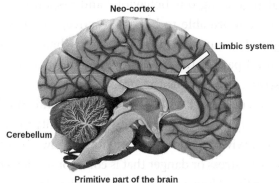

So how does this work on a practical level? Well, potentially what could happen is that the information comes in from either the outside of a person's world, that is the environment, or from the inside world in the form of thoughts and physiological responses, and is processed in the lower part of the brain. Say, for example, someone cuts you up in their car and makes you hit the brakes. The lower parts of your brain will send signals to your body to increase your heart rate and change your body posture; the limbic system signals an angry emotional response whilst the neo-cortex filters through the different responses to find the appropriate words and phrases to use.

Due to this sequential and multi-level processing in our brain, we might react from the lower parts of the brain before we have given our more complex part of the brain a chance to process the information and choose an appropriate response, resulting in a reaction to the event, perhaps a hand gesture, or a more aggressive response than we would have liked.

It is important to understand how the brain handles information in order to be sympathetic and understanding of human behaviour and also for us to understand ourselves and the way we react to situations and experiences. You can get tense, feel angry or have a thought and they are all initiated by some form of stimulation which is being processed in different parts of your brain. As our brains become more mature through the normal process of child development, our neo-cortex begins to help us to regulate the more primitive and reactive areas of our brain, for example impulsivity and frustration, and we get better at regulating our behaviour and responses. Hopefully, we will become more able to be less reactive, less frustrated and more thoughtful in our responses. However, when there is damage to this top-level part of the brain, for example caused by chronic traumatic stress, it increases the probability that this person will have more difficulties in regulating themselves and could increase that individual's aggression, impulsivity, and capacity to be violent.

One of the survival instincts that you might know a bit more about is the response to stress or danger that is commonly referred to as the fight or flight reflex. However, what might be less familiar is the fact that there are a couple of different ways to respond to a perceived threat and these two ways of responding exist on a spectrum and either or both could be recruited, depending on a person's gender, age and other circumstances.

Hyper arousal is the state you'll be in when the signals sent from the brain to the body get you ready for fleeing or fighting. You become impulsive and hyper vigilant, your heart rate increases and your muscles tense. The brain is continuously receiving input from the world outside as well as internal signals. We make a decision as to whether we could stay and fight or run as fast as we can. If we're in a group, we will try and affiliate with others but this state of hyper arousal could also lead to panic, leaving us frozen and unable to act.

On the other side of the spectrum we find something called dissociative adaptation and this is used when your brain is receiving signals that are telling you that you're not going to be able to get away from the situation or fight your way out. Instead, the brain starts to prepare you for injury or pain and to protect you from having to experience this, the brain disengages and withdraws the conscious mind from the world. The person's heart rate slows down; circulation decreases. The person will experience a sense of suspension of time, become more compliant, and have a feeling of numbness and perhaps even faint.

There are, of course, different factors that will determine the response. For example, if you are an adult, you are more likely to be able to flee or perhaps even stay and fight. However, if you're an infant or a child, your only response might be to try and alert someone who can help you by crying or screaming. If there are no options to get away from the situation, the response to the threat and danger will be to dissociate. As the response moves across a spectrum, sometimes in the hyper arousal state and other times in a dissociative state, two people going through the exact same situation will remember different things about that event.

Our nervous system is a very complex system working in our brain, all within neurons and neuron pathways that send signals according to the stimulation that is coming in from outside and inside the body. These systems of neurons will respond in the same way when receiving input that is predictable, moderate and controlled. If there are changes in the stimulation of the system, say for example an increase of input, as long as the input is continuous and non-stop, the tolerance to the input will increase and, in the end, the system will give less of a response. This is often true for people who take certain medication on a regular basis which in the end doesn't work as well because the neurons have adapted to the stimulation of the medication. In some ways, this is a good thing as it allows our network of neurons to be responsive to the environment they are functioning in. Chronic stimulation over a long period of time can make the system almost unresponsive. However, if the system of neurons is subjected to stimulation that is intense and unpredictable, with different timings and intensity, the system instead has the potential to become more sensitive. Any tiny stimulation that would previously cause a small response can instead lead to an extreme activation of the nervous system. The whole system that is there to protect us from threat and danger is put on a constant high alert and becomes vulnerable.

We now know that individuals who grow up in threatening, unpredictable environments, those children and adults who are exposed to neglect and abuse, have a different baseline of alarm compared to others. Their brains tell them that they are under attack even when there is no apparent threat or danger. This means they will think differently, they will function differently and they will behave differently.

Judith Herman (1997, p.99) eloquently describes this:

Adaptation to this climate of constant danger requires a state of constant alertness. Children in an abusive environment develop extraordinary abilities to scan for warning signs of attack. They become minutely attuned to their abusers' inner states. They learn to recognize subtle changes in facial expression, voice, and body language as signals of anger, sexual arousal, intoxication, or dissociation. This nonverbal communication becomes highly automatic and occurs for the most part outside of conscious awareness. Child victims learn to respond without being able to name or identify the danger signals that evoked their alarm.

Many women who are survivors of childhood sexual abuse as well as sexual violence as adults will potentially have a nervous system that is constantly on high alert which means they will often appear fearful, nervous and mistrusting. Their behaviour often comes from an unconscious place and their nervous system is responding instinctually to conditions around and inside them.

Overview of research on pregnancy

Pregnancy can be a challenging and scary time for many women and especially for women who are expecting their first child. Unfortunately, we live in a world where childbirth is often depicted as something that is dangerous and is often compared to the worst pain a woman will ever experience in her life. In reality, there is nothing in life that is 100 per cent safe and anything we do could potentially be dangerous. In my experience, there is a lack of knowledge about physiological birth amongst the general population, and unfortunately also amongst some health professionals. This is not helped by clinical guidelines and policies that rarely protect the physiological process of childbirth.

Many women will have concerns not only about the health and wellbeing of their baby and the experience of labour and childbirth but also about any medical procedures they might encounter. We all get to read the headlines about unnecessary caesareans in the papers as well as hear stories about episiotomies and vaginal tears that never heal. On top of all that, there are a number of pregnancy-related illnesses that some women will experience whilst those often referred to as 'the lucky ones' sail through pregnancy free of any ailments or complications.

So what is it like to be pregnant as a survivor of sexual abuse? We know from studies carried out that women who report being survivors of sexual abuse have a statistically significant higher number of complications during pregnancy, such as bleeding, severe vomiting, accidents, infectious diseases and severe illness (Yampolsky, Lev-Wiesel and Ben-Zion 2010; Lukasse *et al.* 2012).

Survivors of abuse are much more likely to become hospitalised during pregnancy, often due to premature contractions as well as premature birth. It was also noted that survivors were more likely to experience further abuse during their pregnancy, arrange more unscheduled appointments with their antenatal clinics and have a higher number of ultrasound examinations during their first pregnancy, compared to women who had not experienced abuse (Leeners *et al.* 2010).

We can see similar findings in a sample of 357 first-time mothers of whom 37 per cent reported being survivors of sexual abuse before the age of 18. The survivors had 'significantly higher levels of depressive symptomatology, negative life events, and physical and verbal abuse before and during pregnancy' (Benedict *et al.* 1999).

Another study showed similar findings as survivors reported several health complications and a tendency for higher use of heath care services during their pregnancy. This study also concluded that even though survivors report more complications during their pregnancy, it is worth paying attention to the observations that women who are survivors do not experience more obstetric complications during pregnancy and birth compared to women in general (Grimstad and Schei 1999).

Psychologically, survivors of abuse may show more stress and anxiety during pregnancy and have an increase in suicidal thoughts. Survivors may become hyper vigilant and be aware of every sensation in their body, often understanding these signs as danger or trouble, which creates increased worry. Other survivors will be completely unaware of their body and any signals and sensations, which could lead to them not contacting or seeking advice from health professionals for potential obstetric complications (Leeners *et al.* 2006). This is all linked to a nervous system that has become damaged from the trauma and I will talk about this in more detail later on.

One interesting point in this study was that it indicated that many women with an abuse history found childbirth classes frightening as the very thought of lying down among people they'd met for the first time to practise relaxation felt totally unacceptable to them. They did not feel that they would be safe enough to be able to relax. This could potentially mean that many survivors will avoid free or paid-for antenatal classes as they would not want to be asked to practise relaxing. I think this is something that antenatal teachers and providers should take into consideration so that all women can feel welcome and able to attend antenatal classes.

It might be worth mentioning here that talking to survivors antenatally about 'listening to your body' and 'trusting your instincts' might not be very helpful. Survivors often feel like their body has let them down and they have learnt to disconnect from the messages their body is sending them. It might also be very difficult for survivors to trust any instincts as in the past; this might have caused them harm. I'd like to add that many women, survivors or not, are quite disconnected from their bodies, a sign of our times, so it can be a challenge for the majority of women to connect with their body and instincts. We often hear birth professionals telling women these things and it is not until we become aware of the damage these statements can make that we can start to find new ways of communication.

We know that women with a history of sexual abuse more often experience depression, both in the prenatal and postnatal period, compared to women who have not been sexually abused (Spinelli 1997). However, pregnancy can often be a time when women are able to find the space and time to open up and it could be a good time to seek help to process and heal from past trauma. Studies showed that psychotherapy during pregnancy was much more effective than standard parenting programmes in helping women with depression in pregnancy make choices for themselves (Spinelli *et al.* 2016).

Ebony speaks about this:

'As an abuse survivor, I have suffered with depression and anxiety. During my pregnancy, my depression became severe (I never thought pregnancy would affect me so much as a survivor). I was very anxious about my care and treatment during labour and definitely thought my history would affect the labour and birth. I was most scared that the midwife or doctor would be unkind or unsympathetic despite having a wonderful doula. I was terrified of birthing on a labour ward as I didn't want to go through what I perceived would be traumatic interventions.'

We know that a large number of women are fearful of birth and we see this from the steady increase in tocophobia since the beginning of the twenty-first century (O'Connell *et al.* 2017). Again, in survivors we see that this is more prevalent and a Norwegian study, that included 2365 pregnant women, found that a history of sexual abuse significantly increased the risk of having a severe fear of childbirth among first-time mothers. What was quite sad to read in this study was that in women who had already given birth, fear was more associated with a previously traumatic birth experience (Lukasse *et al.* 2009).

It is, of course, not just the fear of childbirth itself that survivors have but also the fear of medical procedures, especially vaginal examinations (VEs). Studies show that 43.5 per cent of women who are survivors of sexual abuse experienced memories from their past abuse during gynaecologic examinations (Leeners *et al.* 2007). I feel this kind of information is vital for anyone who carries out VEs so that they fully understand that they could potentially put someone back in a situation of experiencing sexual abuse.

A survivor often worries that care providers will somehow notice from an examination that she is a survivor, even though there may be no scars or physical signs. Many survivors express a worry that the damage will be imprinted on them somehow, like they've got it written all across their forehead.

Survivors also worry about being touched without being asked first and worry about loss of control. They might also be concerned about the sex of their baby and worry about giving birth to an abuser or someone who could be abused.

Overview of research on childbirth

We have to accept that women who have experienced trauma previously in their lives are more vulnerable during childbirth and that is why everyone must be better educated in providing compassionate and kind support. It simply is not enough to look at good outcomes as equalling a baby and mother that are both alive. This is, of course, very important but the impact on the woman, the baby and the whole family, of how the woman is made to feel during childbirth, has long-lasting effects. The difficulties with bonding that can occur after a traumatic birth will affect that child for a lifetime. The rest of that woman's life is impacted if she carries guilt, believing that she should have known better or blaming herself for what happened during the birth. We cannot allow women to enter maternity services as healthy and strong women and then come out the other side damaged and disempowered or, even worse, women who are already traumatised to become even more damaged. The rippling effects of a traumatic birth experience are far reaching, like a mini tsunami that causes damage to relationships across the board as well as impact on our society.

A study that is worth taking note of took place in Atlanta, USA, with some quite shocking results. In this study, 103 women were interviewed four weeks after giving birth and it concluded that survivors of sexual abuse were 12 times more likely to experience childbirth as a traumatic event (Soet, Brack and Dilorio 2003). That makes for harrowing reading and this is a strong indication that finding out about a woman's previous history makes a lot of sense and potentially prevents further trauma. I think we all must get better at letting women know that, as survivors, when it comes to childbirth, asking for more help and letting care providers know could prevent re-traumatisation. We must make it easier for women to feel able to disclose their past history. This would, of course, not help those survivors who are unaware of their abuse but we need to start somewhere.

A Slovenian doctor, Tanja Repi (2008), reports that in her clinical practice, many pregnant women who have been sexually abused experience distress and new traumas in situations where women without a history of sexual abuse would not have that experience and, if they did, it would be to a much lesser degree.

There might be additional reasons for experiencing distress and trauma beside pain; however, in Finland, a researcher carried out an experimental study which showed that woman with a fear of childbirth have a reduced level of pain tolerance during and after pregnancy when compared to women who had no fear of childbirth (Saisto *et al.* 2001).

Those of us who are familiar with birth physiology will understand that being fearful and full of 'fight or flight' hormones will inhibit the body's natural pain management system for labour. In a physiological birth, the woman will release oxytocin as well as beta-endorphins and both of these hormones help with pain management. If adrenaline is being released it will inhibit release of both of these hormones. It makes total sense that women fearful of birth would experience the whole event as more traumatic and painful.

When a study looked at women referred to counselling for a fear of childbirth it was found that 63 per cent of them were survivors of abuse (Nerum *et al.* 2006). This is not the only study that found a connection between fear of childbirth and abuse. Another study, by Heimstad *et al.* (2006), reported a significant association between tocophobia and sexual and physical abuse in childhood. What was also discovered in this study was that only half of women who report having an experience of physical and sexual abuse in childhood had a vaginal delivery without complications, as opposed to 75 per cent of non-abused women.

Another study found that women with a history of rape are more likely to have elective caesarean births as well as induced labours (Henriksen *et al.* 2014).

In a study carried out by Tallman and Hering, women with no history of sexual abuse were compared to women with such a history and it showed that survivors were significantly more likely to transfer to hospital due to complications. First-time mothers who were also survivors had an increase in caesarean births while all of the women who were survivors used more pharmaceutical pain medication (Tallman and Hering 1998).

However, this study is contradicted by the findings of Benedict *et al.* (1999) who interviewed 357 women and found no significant associations between sexual abuse in the past and mode of birthing and newborn outcomes.

Another study looked at labour outcomes for women who were childhood sexual abuse survivors and women who had been raped in adulthood, compared to a control group. This study showed a significantly higher rate of caesarean and operative vaginal births for women who had been raped in adulthood compared to the other two groups. Their labours were also longer. There were no noticeable differences between the childhood sexual abuse survivors and the control group (Nerum *et al.* 2013).

It's not unusual for a woman with a history of sexual abuse to start feeling as though she no longer has control over her body as the contractions of labour become stronger and more intense. These feelings of losing control can be similar to the feelings she had when the abuse took place. Generally, when you talk to women about what their greatest concerns are with regard to labour and birth, they will often state that it's the perceived loss of control that scares them the most. For a survivor of abuse, these feelings of loss of control can be closely associated with being in a situation where she is not emotionally or even physically safe.

To prevent this from happening, it is extremely important that she is given as much information as possible during labour: what is likely to happen, what it will look like and what is normal and to be expected. This is when a really well-structured antenatal course or a committed healthcare provider who takes the time to explain everything in as much detail as possible throughout labour and birth will make a huge difference. The trauma from the past means that many survivors are programmed to believe that the only way to be safe is to be on constant alert. If a survivor is given a really good explanation of what to expect, this will essentially give her a break from the constant need for control and worry. It will stop her from feeling like a sitting duck, waiting for what may come, unexpectedly and at any time. When survivors feel like this, vulnerable and in immediate danger, studies show that they may resort to extreme behaviour such as aggression, or the complete opposite, submission (Smith 1998). Neither of these behaviours will be helpful for anyone but least of all for the woman in labour.

Esme tries to explain how she felt during the labour and birth of her first baby:

> 'My first labour was very traumatic and I still have no idea how things could have been done differently. The doctor had to apologise to me the next day for shouting at me. They cut my baby's head with the forceps and were very very rough with me. The episiotomy left my husband in tears and the birth scared the on-duty midwives and my mum. I went into complete shock whilst trying to deliver and was shouted at to do better whilst being yanked off a bed by forceps.'

I've been talking here about women who are aware of their abuse history but we know that not all women have this awareness. Studies show that many victims of abuse go into a 'freeze' state and this is a way for the subconscious mind to protect the person from permanent damage (Heidt *et al.* 2005; Möller *et al.* 2017). The brain basically helps the person to survive a difficult event by going somewhere else or dissociating. Even though there is no conscious memory of the abuse, the woman's body still remembers and the unprocessed feelings, such as fear, shame, disgust and also powerlessness can re-surface during childbirth and connect the sensations of labour with the previous abuse. This means that survivors sometimes do the same thing in labour, dissociate from the pain. To some care providers, it might look like the woman is managing fine when her mind has gone elsewhere. It is important to check in with women in labour all the time to discover how they are coping. Calling them by their name and asking them a simple question such as: 'What went through your mind during that contraction?' could be helpful in identifying whether the woman is truly present or not.

Physiological childbirth naturally takes women off to another level of consciousness and women often talk about being on 'planet birth'. The difference is that they are still present in the room while a woman who dissociates might feel like she's on the ceiling, looking down at herself or that she's been disconnected from everyone and everything in the room. This is a time when it would be very helpful for someone to know about a woman's past history, especially if she is a survivor, as that person can remind the woman that this is not abuse, remind her that she is having a baby and explain that memories have been triggered but that the situation is different. The woman needs to know that she is safe.

It might be easy to jump to the conclusion that if the pain of labour and childbirth is removed, the survivor will not dissociate and they will have an easier time. Unfortunately this is not a guarantee for a trauma-free experience. For some women, the use of anaesthesia will be helpful, but for others, the feeling of loss of control could make it more challenging.

Often, the survivor of abuse had no one there just for them, no one who was looking out for them and caring for them. One of the most helpful things for a survivor is to have someone there, like a doula, who is not part of the medical team, not part of the family but who knows about the woman's past history. This person needs to understand and have the knowledge of why a survivor might behave in the way she is and reassure the woman that all is good and she is safe.

Overview of research on the postnatal period

The majority of women are apprehensive about becoming mothers and also want to do the very best they can to protect and care for their child. There is so much pressure on women to be 'perfect' mothers and in my experience and from what I have witnessed, there is little support available, which leads to many women struggling in the postnatal period. I would say that every woman worries about what kind of mother she will be but for women who are survivors, it can be even more intense. Survivors don't only worry about what kind of parents they will be, they also wonder about what actually happens in a 'normal' family and whether what they have been through will impact on their children.

The first time a new mum meets her baby is usually straight after birth when the baby is put skin-to-skin. The sensations of having the baby's body on her skin, along with the baby perhaps trying to latch on can bring up strong feelings. The sensations of having a baby suckle on the breast have the potential to awaken memories of abuse, especially for the survivor who had her breasts groped. If a woman shows an initial strong dislike of breastfeeding, it's very important that no additional pressure is put upon her by well-meaning care providers. What she needs is to be heard and respected and support given when the time is right.

Breastfeeding during the night-time might be especially challenging as this might have been when the abuse happened. Finding creative solutions, like expressing during the day and having someone else feed the baby during the night, might be a way around it.

Some survivors will find it more difficult to breastfeed a son compared to a daughter, especially if their abuser was a man. Other women believe that somehow their milk is 'dirty' because of what happened to them and feel it's best not to expose their newborn to it.

There are not many studies that have looked at survivors of abuse and breastfeeding; however, I discovered a couple of studies. One study found that when comparing women who reported being survivors of childhood sexual abuse to women with no history of abuse, the survivors were 2.6 times more likely to initiate breastfeeding

(Prentice *et al.* 2002). The second study from 1994 found that survivors had 13 per cent higher intentions of breastfeeding their babies compared to their non-abused counterparts (Benedict, Paine and Paine 1994). A recent study from 2017 found that survivors of abuse often reported more frequent problems with breastfeeding, such as mastitis and pain. It was also noted that 20 per cent of women who were survivors of CSA found breastfeeding to be a trigger for their past abuse (Elfgen *et al.* 2017). Another study concluded that women who were survivors of abuse breastfed for as long as women who reported not being survivors (Coles, Anderson and Loxton 2016).

There are a number of things that make the first few months as a new mother overwhelming. No woman can fully prepare for the impact of sleepless nights, hormonal changes, heightened sensitivity and just getting used to looking after a newborn who requires attention around the clock. Women are often told to trust their body as well as their intuition and find it difficult to do so; however, for a sexual abuse survivor, this can be even harder. Trying to figure out what her crying baby needs and feeling like a failure, together with strong feelings of shame, guilt and anxiety often lead to a difficult postnatal period for many.

Numerous studies confirm that survivors of abuse have an increased risk of depression across their life-span. A review of 43 studies carried out recently found that women who were childhood abuse survivors or had been abused by their partners had more lifetime depression and more depression during pregnancy and postnatally (Alvarez-Segura *et al.* 2014). An older study shows that survivors of abuse are four times more likely to develop depression compared to adults who are not survivors (Briere and Elliot 1994).

Some survivors who have grown up in an environment where there was no safety, no family life and things were generally chaotic might want to do everything 'right' as a mother, which often leads to perfectionism. The child's needs are put above everything else and there is a selfless devotion to be a perfect mother. A qualitative study by Berman *et al.* (2014) discovered the challenging process that survivors go through when they become mothers and the deep desire these women have to do things differently in their family. The study found that the women showed great resourcefulness and courage in trying to be the idealised version of what society considers a good mother whilst often struggling with what the realities of motherhood really are as well as their own personal circumstances to provide all that they wanted to for their children.

It has been highlighted in studies that female survivors of CSA displayed some particular traits as parents. They often found difficulties in setting clear boundaries between parent and child and they tended to favour two extreme parenting styles which were in complete contrast. These styles were found to be either permissive parenting or the use of harsh physical discipline (Ruscio 2001).

Many women who are aware that they have been sexually abused worry that they will themselves become abusers of their own children. The fact that the mother has these fears acts as a kind of safeguard and means it is quite unlikely that she will. However, research suggests that it appears that around one-third of abuse survivors will subject their own children to abuse. This figure is around six times higher than the base rate in the general population; the authors rightly argued that a history of abuse is only one of many possible reasons for why this happens (Kaufman and Zigler 1987).

However, there is research out there that has identified three protective mechanisms or factors that prevent women who are survivors from abusing their own children. They are: getting emotional support from at least one non-abusive adult during childhood, the participation in therapy at some point, and a stable, satisfying relationship as an adult.

The conclusion of these studies was that women who experienced one or more of these protective factors did not repeat the cycle of abuse (Egeland, Jacobvitz and Sroufe 1988; Zuravin, McMillen, DePanfilis and Risley-Curtiss 1996).

A more recent study concluded that in a minority of male survivors there may be a risk factor that the abused become the abuser but among the female survivors of abuse there was no correlation (Glasser *et al.* 2001).

What most survivors worry about are the normal tasks associated with parenting, such as changing nappies and other intimate duties.

This causes more stress for survivors as they not only worry about their own boundaries but also worry what others might be thinking about their parenting (Douglas 2000).

The needs of birthing women

While writing a book about how to support survivors of sexual abuse during pregnancy, labour and the postnatal period, I often find it frustrating to think about the fact that these are important needs for all birthing women and if these suggestions were followed, it would make a huge difference to *all* birthing women but especially to those women who are survivors. It's a very personal choice for women where they have their baby, who they choose to be their care providers and so are their choices around medical interventions and pain medication. These choices can be very difficult for most women as it's not easy to imagine what childbirth will be like. For survivors, it might be most important to focus on where they would feel safest and with whom, rather than anything else. This might be true for all women but survivors especially need to protect themselves from their past abuse tainting their birth experience.

Since the birth of obstetrics and modern medicine, pregnancy and childbirth have become safer for many women and their babies. Good care is often associated with modern facilities with access to the latest technology for those of us who live in countries where this is available or have the money to pay for it. This is, of course, great news for the human race; however, with these developments and the rise of technology, we seem to have turned our backs on some of the most important practices when it comes to facilitating childbirth. Physiological processes, like childbirth, happen to us with the help of hormones and, generally, we need to shut down our neo-cortex or 'thinking brain'. Women need to feel safe and secure, warm and loved to support the release of oxytocin, endorphins and all the other hormones needed.

We know from studies that women will remember their birth experiences for the rest of their lives and their strongest memory will be the care they received from their caregivers (Takehara *et al.* 2014). Penny Simkin (1991) suggests in her study that as the woman will remember her caregivers forever, they should bear in the forefront of their mind: 'How will she remember this?' This is something very easy and practical that we all can apply to our reflective practice.

A study in Iceland identified three main areas of need for women during childbirth and those were: (1) caring and understanding from their attendants; (2) security, which involved being kept informed of what was happening; and (3) a sense of control of self and circumstances (Halldórsdóttir and Karlsdóttir 1996).

Caring and understanding from attendants

Caring and understanding from the people who are supporting the woman has been shown to be extremely important in numerous studies and, in all honesty, I don't think we need studies to confirm that fact. Women have always needed and looked for support in labour from kind and empathetic caregivers. Many women now look to doulas for the emotional and practical support which I would say is mainly due to the current state of maternity services in many countries. It's not that midwives can't or won't provide this kind of support but usually they simply don't have the time as their focus is often on record keeping. It certainly doesn't help either that most maternity units are short staffed and, overall, we have a shortage of midwives in England (RCM 2017).

A large-scale review of the research available by Cochrane concluded that continuous support from someone who was not part of the hospital care team or the woman's family improved the outcome for both the mother and the baby. This person should have some training as well as experience of providing emotional and practical support and the authors suggested that this person should be a doula (Bohren *et al.* 2017).

As care providers, working with survivors, we need to understand that memories of their abuse could re-emerge at any time during pregnancy and childbirth, and be prepared for this. As has been mentioned, the woman may not have any memories at all of the abuse, especially if it was during her childhood, and triggers and events during your meetings with her or during birth could bring extremely strong emotions to the surface. Survivors may act and behave in ways which they did with their abuser, become submissive, without a voice, or not showing any signs of wanting to make choices or become 'difficult'; they may be mistrusting, questioning everything that is being suggested and even become angry and aggressive.

It's well documented by Penny Simkin that patients who are referred to as 'difficult' or 'awkward' have often been through some type of trauma. Anyone with PTSD who has not had any treatment for their condition will often react to stressful situations by either switching off and dissociating or having a panic attack or hyper arousal of their nervous system. It's worth mentioning here that I believe many maternity workers could possibly have PTSD and not receive treatment for this condition. Potentially, this means there are a lot of people working in the system without the capability to assess situations from a clear and healthy mind. There needs to be more support available for those who care for others.

Security and being kept informed

Halldórsdóttir and Karlsdóttir's (1996) research showed that a feeling of security, which included being kept informed about what was happening during labour, was important to women during childbirth. Informed choice and the acceptance and support of those choices by caregivers will go a very long way. Assisting and making sure that the information is given in a straightforward and objective way will help women make those choices. The majority of guidelines for medical professionals clearly state that if a medical procedure needs to be carried out, the information should be given to the woman beforehand. This information should include any risks associated with the procedure and any possible alternatives, as well as what the risks could be if nothing is done. I will talk further about this in Chapter 3 when I discuss consent and human rights.

What I've seen sometimes is that medical professionals hide some of the information from the women in labour and their birth partner too and I believe this is done partly to prevent them from worrying about what is going to happen and also because it is easier to simply give the information which is needed in the moment rather than a running commentary of what is happening and the possible outcomes. It might be a better strategy to work as a team and explain to everyone involved what is being discussed and considered outside of the birthing room. Keeping women and their partners 'in the dark' usually leads to dissatisfaction with the birth experience and extra work down the line.

Something that is very important is that every time someone enters the birthing room, that person should introduce themselves and talk to the woman and her partner before starting to look at any machines or notes. Making someone feel like they are part of the furniture or less important than a machine can do so much damage.

A sense of control of self and circumstances

I often hear women talking about wanting to be in control of their birthing experience and have over the years come to realise that it's not just control over their own behaviour in labour that they mean, but also being in control of what is done to them by others as well as being in control of what their own body is doing. It might be worth exploring with women what their exact worries are around loss of control. It can be easy to assume that all women worry about the same things but that is often not the case. By asking questions to clarify what women mean when they say they want to be in control will be helpful in knowing how to support them better.

For survivors, being in control is extremely important as any feelings of being unheard, helpless or out of control usually have an association with the abuse they endured. All women need to feel that they have an equal part in the decision-making and that they are involved in all decisions around their care. It's extremely important that informed consent is given before anything is done to a woman in labour, especially survivors.

It could be very helpful for women to learn about what to expect in labour, potential triggers and what the different medical procedures involve. For example, a woman having a caesarean birth might not be aware that her vagina will be touched and that swabs will be inserted to mop up any blood loss. She will most likely also have a catheter to collect urine, and a suppository inserted for pain relief, which involves touching her in areas where she might assume she won't be touched. This is something that was concerning to Anna:

> 'I'm also gravely aware that women having caesarean births often have their vagina touched for a catheter and other things. I never would have known this and there's evidence to suggest the body has a memory. If you're a survivor and then you have a caesarean, which is abdicating control as it is, then to not know your vagina has been touched during the procedure but for things to feel different must be so confusing to a woman, it would be to me.'

If a woman notices that someone has touched her but she was not told, she might wonder what happened to her. For a survivor, this could make her feel like she's been abused again and the body does remember what has been touched and interfered with.

Understanding what a normal physiological birth might look like, the sounds women make and the way their body is working is extremely helpful. Simkin and Klaus (2004) talk about rehearsing some of the sounds and movements with women before birth which could make it more normal and desensitise women. They also suggest talking to women about what they consider unacceptable behaviour and acceptable behaviour. This would help them feel more in control of what their body might do in labour and birth.

Chapter 2

Working with Survivors

Pregnancy and Birth

Impact of sexual abuse on pregnancy

Many survivors of sexual abuse will lead completely normal and successful lives and being a survivor doesn't necessarily mean that someone will have all of the issues and behaviours discussed in this book. At the same time, many women can display some or many of these symptoms but that doesn't necessarily mean that they are survivors of abuse. However, it might be a good idea to assume that many women in your care will have been sexually harassed or abused at some point in their lives. I say this as, in my experience, the majority of women feel vulnerable as they give birth to their child. Birth physiology depends largely on the environment and the way women are made to feel by their caregivers. Every woman in labour should be treated with kindness, dignity and respect.

It is, understandably, difficult to say exactly how sexual abuse impacts on the abused person as it will have influenced everything in that person's life: the way the woman feels about her body, about becoming a parent, relationships, trust, mental health, self-confidence, etc. Some of the consequences might not be apparent until they are triggered or awakened again by a situation or experience which is similar to the abuse.

The majority of women I speak to have no idea that the abuse and trauma they were subjected to in their past would have an impact on their pregnancy and birth. They simply do not put the two together, which is understandable. Sue explains that she had no idea of how the sexual abuse she suffered at the hands of her father would affect her pregnancy:

'I was totally unprepared for everything that being pregnant would bring up. It would be the start of a whole range of emotions and experiences that looking back on now, I would not wish to happen to any other woman. I can look back at this time so much differently now and I can grasp why what happened to me had such a huge impact on my pregnancy. I never attended any antenatal classes as I felt I didn't fit in. I have always been very resilient and just thought that I didn't need anyone. I could do this on my own!'

Georgia, who was raped, explains:

'Before getting pregnant I never thought that it could impact me. And even when I found out that I was pregnant it didn't even occur to me. However during my pregnancy I saw something on Instagram which was a workshop for pregnant women who were also survivors of sexual abuse. This made me think about it and actually become quite paranoid that it would suddenly affect me.'

Holly didn't think that the abuse by a friend of her granddad would impact on her future and, like many survivors, she felt she should just 'get on with it'.

'To be honest, I was too young at the time to think about how it might affect my future. I got pregnant when I was 18 and even then I knew that I was not comfortable with anyone seeing me give birth but I just got on with it. I had told my partner but I don't think he even realised that the two things might affect each other; if he did he never said anything to me.'

Leila, who was in an abusive relationship as a young woman, was asked by her midwife during an antenatal appointment whether she had experienced sexual abuse in her past and she was also told that it could have an impact on her birth experience.

'I had totally forgotten that I had been asked the question. In fact, I think I had forgotten this pretty soon after she had asked. It just didn't feel relevant. I didn't see how it would affect me and just assumed that there are people who have been through far worse so could totally understand why issues may potentially arise.'

Pregnancy is a time in a woman's life when she should be able to enjoy her changing body, feel excitement about meeting her baby and starting a family of her own. Pregnancy can also be a time for memories of a woman's own childhood to re-surface and for survivors of abuse these can bring thoughts of worry about what kind of parents they will be. Being pregnant can feel like losing control of what is happening to the woman's body and even bring thoughts about the growing foetus taking over or invading her body. If the woman knows she's expecting a boy, she might even feel repulsed about the fact that she has a penis growing inside of her. There might even be a strong desire to terminate the pregnancy.

On a positive note, not all survivors have negative feelings surrounding the pregnancy and some will, instead, feel empowered and strong during pregnancy, feeling that their bodies are finally doing something right. Georgia explains this:

'During my pregnancy I actually felt very present in my body for the first time. In a wonderful way. Very grateful and very confident and in awe of my body. I really loved my body which was so positive. It was the first time in my life.'

On the other hand, many survivors, when deciding to start a family, can have fertility problems, perhaps due to infections or damage caused by the abuse, and may also suffer from multiple miscarriages. Many survivors also believe that their body has been damaged and can no longer perform normal tasks, like carrying a baby. Sue, who was unable to tell anyone about her father's abuse, despite numerous hospital admissions for different problems, shares her thoughts:

'I had many hospital visits with various symptoms. I was a school refuser and can clearly remember being dragged to school, only to walk straight out. I was threatened by so-called professionals telling me that I was out of control, with one female doctor saying I would never be able to have children due to my behaviour.'

It's not unusual for survivors to have exaggerated symptoms of pregnancy, such as hyperemesis gravidarum, hypertension, fatigue, heartburn, joint pains, backache, Braxton-Hicks contractions, sleeplessness, constipation and more (Simkin and Klaus 2004). Some of these things might be due to psychosocial as well as medical reasons so it's always a good idea for health professionals to take a holistic approach rather than treating just the symptoms and not the cause. Sharon believes that the worry about her unborn child during pregnancy led to some of her pregnancy symptoms:

'For me it was the anxious feeling of wanting to protect my child from ever experiencing what I had. The anxiety caused more sickness and sleepless nights.'

What most survivors worry about is the upcoming birth and the invasive procedures that they might be subjected to. There are fears around the pain of childbirth and the damage to their bodies from bringing their baby into the world.

Gita felt that she was not given adequate information, which would have reassured her and made her feel more in control leading up to the birth of her baby.

'Not knowing I had choices around many aspects of pregnancy care e.g. I didn't know I didn't have to go to scans that I found

uncomfortable. When I researched and discovered I didn't have to have a doppler listening in during labour...[the] midwife then told me they could use a pinard during antenatal visits too. I understand midwifery care is stretched...and I feel following standard procedure and not explaining choices available is withholding valuable information that creates true informed consent.'

One of the main concerns for survivors is, understandably, the VEs that take place during labour and sometimes in pregnancy. It could be the case that the association with touch to this part of the woman's body is to feel numb or to feel that someone is trying to control her (Zoldbrod 2015). The thought of strangers touching and 'poking' around can bring up very strong feelings. Shanay explains how it made her feel when she found out that this was part of routine care in childbirth:

'Being told that part of the normal procedure of labour was vaginal finger insertions to see how many centimetres wide I was dilated. As someone who fears my own fingers and my own husband's fingers entering my vagina, being told that this was the only way, was frightening to me. I feared labour so much because of this.'

Midwives and doulas will know that there are other signs of progress in labour, such as the sounds the woman is making, the way she focuses on what is going on in her body, turning inwards and how often and how long the contractions are lasting. There are also external signs, such as the baby moving down in the pelvis, spontaneous rupture of membranes (SROM), a dark line appearing at the onset of the second stage of labour, running from the anal margin and extending between the buttocks, as well as the Rhombus of Michaelis, a kite-shaped area in the back which extends and moves outwards at the beginning of the second stage of labour.

In fact, VEs are currently the 'gold standard' to assess cervical dilation during labour; however, as one study showed, carried out on realistic soft cervical models, only 19 per cent of cervical dilatation measurements were accurate (Huhn and Brost 2004). This is a rather shocking statistic when you consider that decisions on what to do next in terms of interventions are often based on these examinations and can lead to the familiar 'cascade of interventions', where an intervention, such as artificial rupture of membranes (ARM) and augmentation, leads to the need for further interventions, often due to foetal distress.

Due to her great distress about having strangers' fingers inserted in her vagina, Shanay went looking for more information but found that despite her strong wishes for alternatives, she was not met with approval:

> *'During a course, I discovered that there were other ways of checking how things were going. If you looked at the pregnant woman's back, there was a purple line that appeared which indicated something. I can't really remember. Something like that, but that inserting fingers was not the only way. I asked for this other method several times but perhaps it is not as popular or the staff were not trained in that area, but the fact that it wasn't given real consideration made me feel very disrespected, powerless, insignificant again.'*

This feeling of being disrespected and powerless can be a recurrent theme for many survivors. It's quite simple – they do not feel listened to or heard! When a woman who is a survivor speaks up for herself, asks for information or simply says 'no', she must be respected and acknowledged. Sexual abuse is very much about power and survivors feel like all their power was taken away from them. When a healthcare professional does the same, it repeats the cycle and puts huge dents in that woman's chances of recovery. Paula explains that this felt worse than the VEs:

> *'I found VEs quite unpleasant. Also, being treated like a child when refusing things in advance like vitamin K [injection for the baby]. Oddly I found that even more triggering than VEs*

*from a midwife. The feeling of having to get 'clearance' or
'permission' from a male consultant by my midwives, saying
that telling them 'no thanks' wasn't enough, then them setting up
a special appointment to further discuss it and for me to have to
justify myself, brought back feelings of being too young to make
decisions for myself or have any power over my own body and
choices. I wasn't even in a high-risk bracket so the whole thing
felt ridiculous and disempowering.'*

I was once supporting a woman during an induction of labour and
she was connected to continuous monitoring every four hours.
During one of those monitoring sessions, the midwife came in to
strap the sensors onto my client's tummy. My client was on her back,
semi-reclined and said that it felt uncomfortable, which the midwife
interpreted as being the pain from the contractions my client was
having. The midwife asked if my client wanted pain medication. Once
again, my client asked if she could change position as it was painful
and again, the midwife ignored her and simply said that it wouldn't
be for long. My client started crying and the midwife was completely
surprised and could not understand why she was crying. At this point,
I asked the midwife if it was possible for my client to lie on her side
for the monitoring and the midwife agreed that this position would
work. When she left, my client turned to me and said: 'Why was she
not listening to me? I was raped at college and I felt just like I was
back in that situation, in pain, asking someone to stop and they still
carried on.'

I did not know that my client was a survivor until that moment,
but it showed me how incredibly important it is to pay attention to
what women are saying. At no point did my client give consent for
the monitoring to take place; when she gently tried to say that she was
in an uncomfortable position, she was not listened to which brought
back memories of the rape.

To ask or not to ask

I think it is staggering that more and more is invested in maternal mental health services to deal with Post-traumatic Stress Syndrome (PTSS), PTSD and Postnatal Depression (PND), when surely we should instead invest more in preventing it in the first place. There should be clear guidelines in place for all care providers to ask about previous trauma and refer to a dedicated body within the NHS trust to help women work through any trauma before their baby's birth day. It's not just trauma from sexual abuse; any kind of trauma that has not been dealt with has the potential to heavily impact a woman's mothering journey. This relates not only to the birth experience but also to the woman's experiences afterwards and the way she deals with becoming a mother and bonding with her baby.

This is something Sue feels very strongly about. She has had four children and, despite disclosing being a survivor when pregnant with her third and fourth children, she was never directly asked about it:

> 'We are no nearer now in how these issues need to be addressed than we were 35 years ago. I feel so saddened that there are women going through the pain and shame of their past. Even though it doesn't belong to them. This needs to change. There needs to be much more information, not just a leaflet on a doctor's wall. The impact that this has on society is so great it is like a time bomb. The conversations need to happen, for those women who have yet to speak about their abuse and those who already have. It is a subject that most people would never want to have to even think about, let alone talk about. But if we are going to have the trauma of the past cared for and listened to this has to be put in place.'

There are a number of barriers for survivors as well as for care providers in bringing up the subject of sexual abuse and violence. For many care providers, it can feel overwhelming to ask the women they care for about abuse in the past. Often care providers don't feel well equipped to discuss or support women with these issues and they also worry about doing more damage. Another reason might be that there isn't enough time to bring such a serious topic up without a proper plan on how to proceed and find the appropriate help for them. Most appointments with midwives during pregnancy are only ten minutes long and it could be a worry that bringing these things up could cause the woman to break down, and perhaps do some harm to herself or her baby, ending in the care providers getting into trouble. Sylvia explained that more time would have been really beneficial in the antenatal meetings:

> 'Well, some contact with a midwife that was longer than five minutes might have helped. A conversation about the emotional impact of labour would have been an idea, along the lines of "Some women find being in labour a very emotionally vulnerable time. If there are things in a woman's past that have hurt or scared her, these feelings can be triggered again during childbirth" might have helped me make the connection and perhaps confide in her.'

There are many reasons why survivors find it very difficult to disclose their previous history and these can stop them from doing so. They may feel ashamed and embarrassed about what happened to them and also ashamed of people knowing their secret. Often survivors blame themselves for what happened and think that it was somehow their fault; or they might be fearful of the repercussions of disclosing as it could break up their family, or they might themselves be seen as potential abusers of their own children. Trusting others, especially someone in a position of authority, is a huge challenge for most survivors and they worry about not being believed if they did tell someone. It might even be the case that the survivor is not sure that the care provider can handle the disclosure and that it will make them feel uncomfortable. What is also worth bearing in mind is that the woman might not have any memory of the abuse or might believe that it would not be of any relevance.

Despite the many barriers which make it difficult for survivors to talk about their past, many want someone to ask them about it and believe it would be helpful during pregnancy and childbirth. These women might have from a young age been trying to send out signals and signs to others for help, for someone to notice and ask them about it. Here they are in a new situation where they need to trust someone in a position of authority and they might be hoping that someone will ask the right questions.

Sharon, who was sexually abused by her swimming instructor in full view of her mother, wished that the midwife had asked her more questions:

> *'I wish she would have dug a little deeper about why I was anxious, or why I didn't want to be in hospital.'*

Georgia also wished that her midwife had asked her about her previous trauma or life events:

> *'My midwife never asked me, and I never mentioned it to her. Now that I am thinking about it, I suppose I do wish that they had given me the opportunity to share with them my history, if I had felt safe to do so. I would have actually felt very safe telling them, as I felt safe in their space and around them. I think that it would have been nice to get that out in the open in the beginning so that if anything did come up for me we could have been prepared for that. And I think it would have made me feel less afraid of it affecting me.'*

On the other hand, Holly didn't feel that discussing her past with her care providers would have made a difference; looking back, she's not sure now:

> *'They probably couldn't have done anything differently as I was not ready to tell anyone so I doubt anything that they may or may not have done would have changed that for me. Now when I reflect on it I wish I had said something as they may have been able to help me.'*

If there is a disclosure, it is important that, if further support is offered, it is appropriate support and not just a tick-box exercise. For women who want help, being offered extra support that doesn't meet their needs could prove to be more damaging.

Ebony explains:

'I said I was really struggling with depression in my pregnancy and was referred to a "specialist" midwife. No offence meant but this turned out to be a very young midwife who was covering the position and had no counselling or similar skills. It was completely unhelpful. Although I did disclose my history, the sessions felt pointless (I'd done a lot of therapy privately and had knowledge of what would be helpful). She was kind but it wasn't appropriate support and just made me feel even less understood. I wish there had been an option to tick if support was needed in this area and then proper support given.'

Sue has very strong views on this and she agrees with Ebony:

'If a woman has already disclosed that she is a survivor, I truly believe that there has to be support put in straight away. There will be so many thoughts and feelings going through her head. Just knowing that she has someone that she can turn to at any time will be one of the most valuable things that she can ever have. No harsh medical environments and the least possible amount of medical intervention.'

The problems with asking if someone is a survivor of sexual abuse on a questionnaire is that a woman might tick the box to indicate that she is a survivor and then have no one bring this up or take it any further. I can only imagine the bravery of the woman doing this who is then left with no extra support. This is what happened to Gita when she mentioned in her birth plan that she was a survivor:

'I put "history of sexual assault" on my first child's birth plan. This plan was looked over by many people, including senior midwives, and no one spoke to me about this or questioned if I'd had support.'

The other problem is that the woman won't know who will have access to this paperwork. Who will know and be able to learn about her history if she does tick the box? If a questionnaire is used it's important to explain where this will be filed and who will have access to it; otherwise the woman might deem it safer not to disclose.

A more suitable way to ask women if they are survivors might be to simply do this face to face. It's important if this is what you choose to do that you make clear that all women are asked these questions, as survivors often worry that somehow others will be able to tell that they are survivors, perhaps that somehow it can be seen and observed in their bodies, like it's been written on their forehead. You might want to use a statement to show how common it is and then follow up with a question.

Penny Simkin (Simkin and Klaus 2004) gives the following suggestion:

Many women have had unpleasant sexual experiences – being touched or forced into sex – or they have been physically abused. Have you ever experienced anything like that?

Barbara Wiljma, a Norwegian midwife, suggests the following wording:

Many adult women were abused as children, that is, hit or beaten, shouted at, or forced to do sexual things. Did anything like that ever happen to you or is it happening today?

It's probably most helpful if you can come up with your own way of asking, as the more authentic it sounds, the more likely it is that the survivor will feel able to trust you and answer the question honestly. As a doula, I ask my clients if there is anything that they feel would be important for me to know to help support them better. They might not disclose at the time of me asking but sometimes they will call me later and tell me about previous abuse.

Shanay found it very helpful to be able to tell her midwife who asked her in one of the antenatal appointments:

'We had a very detailed discussion. She was so helpful and understanding. She is the one who insisted that during labour, I have my own room. She also fought for my husband to stay overnight for the whole duration of the labour because I told her that I was afraid of what someone might do to me. When she said that I should be safe, that these people at the hospital are professional, I replied with "You don't know what's in people's hearts. Family are supposed to be trustworthy yet how many people are raped and abused by their own relatives?"'

Melanie, on the other hand, found that no one was willing to provide the space for her to feel safe enough to talk about her stepdad's physical and sexual violence against her as a child:

'Not at any point in my pregnancies or births has any healthcare professional provided a safe opportunity to enable me to disclose, not even during triggering moments, whereby I disassociated, cried or became tricky to deal with nor have they asked directly. I don't believe the current system of care is set up to best support survivors, there isn't a relationship built in order to feel safe to disclose, the lack of continuity of carer fails to support survivors, the thought of constantly repeating your story to every person who you encounter during your pregnancy and birth is overwhelming.'

Paula agrees that not seeing the same midwife or caregiver during pregnancy makes it difficult to build up trust. Paula was never asked during any of her five pregnancies if she was a survivor and she says:

'I never had that kind of rapport with a midwife because I never saw one that I felt happy to confide in, often enough. Continuity of midwife would have made a difference. Domino care with a trusted midwife would have given me the space to build up a relationship and give me the time and space to confide in her. I do wonder if it would've meant more sensitive care at my hospital birth.'

(Domino care is when a woman receives the same antenatal care as for a homebirth, that is, in her home with the local homebirth team, but with a hospital birth planned instead. The midwife she gets to know in the community comes to her house and then comes with her to the hospital during the birth.)

On the other hand, some survivors just aren't ready to discuss or face their past during pregnancy and will often miss many of their antenatal appointments. Sue talks about this:

'I did not disclose during my pregnancy. At the time I had not told anyone what was happening to me. I am not sure if disclosing would have helped me personally at the time as my level of dissociation at the time was very high. I strongly feel that there has to be something in place for these questions to happen. The midwife appointments are too short for this kind of conversation to happen. I also think that there is a fear of having the "CONVERSATION" from professionals. I limited my antenatal appointments to as little as possible.'

In research by Sarah Nelson and Sarah Phillips (2001) they identified the most important aspects that survivors found helpful when disclosing their abuse history. The most helpful person had the following qualities:

- is secure about boundaries, but relates with warmth and kindness
- is informed and aware about CSA, or keen to learn
- has examined his/her own issues around CSA
- works non-hierarchically, consults clients, reaches joint decisions
- is client-centred, flexible, imaginative
- neither hides behind confidentiality, nor breaks it insensitively
- has courage to stay with clients through distressing details or behaviour
- is prepared to work over a period of time, though brief contacts can sometimes be the catalyst to life changes.

In essence, your personal qualities are much more important than your professional qualifications for handling and dealing with a disclosure of sexual abuse. Being a good listener and setting boundaries around what you're able to offer and ensuring you signpost to relevant support do not require specific counselling skills. Accepting and believing what the survivor is telling you will enable them to trust you and together you can work out a way forward.

Part of moving forward is to involve the survivor in what care and support they think they might need. You could ask them what they consider to be the areas they need most help with right now or if there is any problem in particular that they feel the abuse has left them with (Nelson and Phillips 2001).

I think Sue has summed it up in terms of how she felt during her pregnancy and what survivors need from health professionals:

'In an ideal world a survivor would have somebody that they trust and can talk to at any time day or night. For me if I was where I am now in my recovery, I know that I would greatly benefit from this. If I was talking about my 17-year-old self this would be something totally different. I felt ashamed, scared that someone could see what had happened to me. Frightened that my baby would be taken from me. That somehow it was my fault that I had let this happen to me. That I wouldn't be seen to be able to look after my baby. This had to be kept to myself at all costs.'

Summary

- It seems that for survivors to be able to disclose, they need to have the continuous support of someone during their pregnancy that they can start to trust and rely on. It's important to see the same caregiver on a regular basis.
- Talking to all women about how common abuse is and educating them on the fact that, in most cases, it will have an impact on their pregnancy, birth and postnatal experience might make it more likely that women will disclose.

- When a woman discloses to you, make sure this is acknowledged and that you, together with her, talk about how to move forward. This might mean referring to another professional service, such as counselling or trauma treatment.
- Informing her of who will have access to the disclosed information is important. She needs to be able to decide if she wants the information to be shared or not.

How to respond to disclosure

It is incredibly important that you show on every level that you believe the woman when she discloses abuse or sexual violence. If the woman is a CSA survivor, she might have tried to tell someone as a child and not been heard or believed. If she now thinks you do not believe her, this could really damage your continued relationship with her.

It's important to acknowledge what she has told you and perhaps reply that this should not happen to anyone and that you're sorry to hear that it happened to her. Make sure you re-affirm her feelings and let her know that it is natural to have feelings of pain, shame and anger.

It usually isn't necessary for you as a caregiver to know all the details of the abuse so don't ask inappropriate questions and make sure you're guided by her as to how much she wants to disclose to you. If you feel able to and willing to offer her support it's up to you how you proceed. In the past when I've worked with survivors, I would tell them that I would be happy for them to talk to me about it and I would do what I could to support and help them but we would have an agreement that if we arrived at a point where I didn't feel that I was able to help or I felt she needed more qualified support, we would look for that support together. It's important to recognise your own limitations and also ensure that you don't promise more than you are able to give.

You might be in a position where you would like to signpost or refer her to professional support in the form of perinatal mental health support or trauma counselling straightaway. Suggest this to her and come to agreements together. It's important that you don't take charge and make her feel out of control. She needs to be in control of her choices and it's up to her what she wants to do. You might want to explain that many survivors also suffer from PTSD and that this requires specific therapeutic input to help heal some of those symptoms before labour and birth. Usually Cognitive Behaviour Therapy (CBT) is recommended for the treatment of trauma but there is a relatively new form of therapy, Eye Movement Desensitisation and Reprocessing (EMDR), which is proving to make impressive improvements to the lives of PTSD sufferers (e.g. see Zepeda Méndez *et al.* 2018).

Discuss with her the potential impact that previous sexual abuse or sexual violence could have during pregnancy, birth and the postnatal period and how you can work together to help minimise and prevent any further trauma. It's especially relevant to talk about triggers and it's also helpful for survivors to get a really in-depth understanding of what happens during different routine procedures.

Summary

- Believe what she tells you.
- Acknowledge and empathise with her experience.
- Offer your own support or signpost her to other appropriate services.
- Resist the temptation to take charge. It is important to allow her to make her own choices.
- Avoid offering support you can't give, and recognise your limits.

Understanding triggers

Anyone subjected to any kind of trauma will have associated specific cues with the traumatic experience. These might be internal or environmental cues that in some way remind a person about the trauma or recall traumatic memories. These cues are often referred to as triggers and they can be quite self-evident but, at times, also very subtle. It's not always the case that all of the memory from the trauma is triggered; it can be just pieces of it, a feeling or a sensation. It can be very helpful for trauma survivors to be aware of what might trigger their past trauma but also for the people around them so that they can better understand actions and behaviours.

Triggers can be words or actions that might have a double or hidden meaning for a survivor of abuse. They can elicit reactions and responses, which might seem to others to be exaggerated or over the top, and this is due to the direct association that they have with the previous trauma. Triggers are usually different for all women and many women are unaware of what could be potential triggers that can bring back strong memories of the abuse during their pregnancy, labour and birth.

If childbirth becomes a traumatic experience it can be a trigger and bring back memories of any past trauma, including sexual abuse. This can then manifest in the woman through flashbacks and body memory. The most frequent triggers are VEs or other procedures where she feels like she can't get away; even continuous monitoring could be a trigger. Additionally, pain during or after the childbirth itself can be a trigger, particularly if the pain is in the woman's vagina, around her stomach and back, or her breasts. It is often the person who a woman feels she should trust the most during childbirth who can subconsciously remind her of the perpetrator who abused her trust as an authority figure. If this happens to her, the woman then (re)experiences the feelings of powerlessness, humiliation, shame and horror.

In his book, *The Post-Traumatic Stress Disorder Sourcebook,* Schiraldi (2009) describes and lists different types of triggers as follows:

- sensory: similar sights, sounds, smells, tastes, touch, position or pain, nausea, rapid heart rate
- anniversary or significant date
- similar, stressful events
- strong emotions

- related thoughts
- related routines or behaviours
- combinations of the above
- out-of-the-blue (when relaxed or with defences against remembering down).

Many of the challenges survivors face during labour and childbirth are tied up directly to triggers, and that is why they become such big obstacles for the woman. For a woman to give birth physiologically, she needs to be able to trust and respond to her body's signals and feel safe to release and let her baby be born. As birth workers, we understand that if the woman is producing adrenaline it will inhibit the flow of oxytocin and endorphins, the birthing hormones needed for the baby to be born.

Sylvia, who was attacked from behind as she walked home from a night out, remembers what triggered her during labour:

> 'One thing I remember is finally getting into labour land – I had been fiercely holding on and battling my labour, trying to stay in control and "dignified". Knowing what I know now, the midwives had done a great job, switching off the lights and encouraging me to slow dance with my husband. I was just drifting off into that otherworld place of oxytocin-intoxication and someone touched me on my shoulder. It completely freaked me out and my brain was on high alert for a long time after that. I don't think it's surprising that it took me a long time to reach full dilation or that my second stage was three hours long.'

Having people approaching from behind the woman can often present a challenge or act as a trigger. It can be very helpful for someone like an anaesthetist, who will be working behind the woman, to introduce themselves properly, standing in front of the woman, without a mouth guard on. During the procedure of siting an epidural, it would also help to explain the procedure step by step, before the next thing happens, for example, 'You will soon feel a cold liquid on your back, which is iodine to make sure your back is sterile and free of bacteria.' Step-by-step instructions for survivors are particularly helpful.

The place of the bed in relation to the door is also something worth considering. If a woman has her back to the door, she might not feel safe at all. Many survivors live with this on a daily basis, making sure that when in a restaurant, their back is not against the door.

It's so important that everyone who enters the room with a woman in labour always knocks and also introduces themselves. It's a good idea to keep the room as private as possible and avoid staff walking in and out, looking for equipment, such as pinards or thermometers and keys to the drugs cabinet. This is something that I see happening far too much in a hospital setting and, at times, it makes me wonder where the woman-centred care we all want has gone. I'm sure that there can be a way of writing policies that would make all this disturbing of women in labour stop. In my view, this is all part of providing respectful and dignified maternity care.

Holly's experience during the birth of her only child shows how there were a number of things that happened to her which made her feel triggered and also traumatised again:

'I recall it as feeling really helpless, with no support. I was very drugged and exhausted. I had lots of medical students watching my forceps birth; so many that they couldn't shut the theatre door fully. They miscounted the swabs after they had stitched me up and they were talking about having to open me up again to look for it. The local anaesthetic for the episiotomy didn't work and I could feel everything. The doctor complained that I was moving and two midwives had to hold me down. My partner was there but I don't remember him supporting me in any way.'

Not being believed or listened to were recurring themes and triggers for the survivors who helped fill out my questionnaire; these triggers in turn led to feelings of being ignored and made to feel unimportant. Sylvia talks about how she didn't receive enough pain medication for suturing after the birth and how this triggered strong feelings:

'I was put in lithotomy. No one asked my permission. No one explained what was going to happen. The injections hurt beyond words. The gas and air [Entonox] was given to me. The stitching started and it was absolutely agonising – much worse than the birth. This time I didn't disassociate, I spoke up and said it hurt. I was told that it was bound to be a little uncomfortable but that I had the full amount of local anaesthetic and it would be over soon. Whilst memories of my attack weren't triggered at the time, all the same feelings were – fury, fear, pain, disgust and I did make quite a fuss and was told to calm down or the doctor wouldn't be able to do a good job.'

Difficulties with VEs were also a recurrent theme for triggering survivors. Leila remembers being examined by a male obstetrician:

'The VEs by the male consultant triggered bad memories. Whilst I didn't really think about it at the time, I do wonder now – was he rough or was I simply more tense because he was male?'

Gita felt extremely triggered due to a multitude of reasons:

'Vaginal examination and being told what to do and being told I was too loud were triggers for me. I was given an internal examination whilst I was standing up, which I didn't give consent to. It was a very big trigger for me as well as not feeling respected by the staff. My voice not being listened to. Also being told I needed to not bear down (wasn't aware I was) like I no longer knew my own body and needed someone who knew better than me to make judgements for me. I felt intimidated as there were a lot of people in the room at this time. It felt like I couldn't say no, similar to not having a voice whilst being assaulted.'

Another recurrent theme is that of the attitude and responses of those who care for women during labour and birth. Everyone that woman comes in contact with and their actions are extremely important during childbirth.

We can conclude that the body of a survivor of abuse has already been violated in the past, perhaps even had severe pain inflicted on it. This means that the care received from care providers during labour and birth could be adding to the suffering and violation. The survivor might experience what is happening to her in exactly the same way as she experienced the abuse. In addition to this, care providers might also use phrases such as 'try and relax and it will hurt less' or 'lie still and I'll do this quickly', or other such phrases where the same words might have been used by a perpetrator during the abuse. These are all potentially huge triggers for a survivor, which could put them back in their past. A survivor who has a flashback might become rigid and freeze, dissociate from the situation, or become compliant and apathetic, or she might panic.

Flashbacks to previous situations of abuse can be triggered by any kind of touch, even if that touch is loving and gentle. It's not always the case that the perpetrator of abuse was forceful; they could have been gaining trust by making the survivor feel loved and special. This is why we must always ask before we touch a woman in labour and why it makes such a difference if at least one of the care providers with the survivor has met her before to discuss things like touch and massage. We need to make sure we look at the woman and connect with her before touching any part of her body. I believe there is always time to do this and it makes a huge difference.

Paula explains how not being heard made her feel and how being touched by people triggered her in labour:

> 'Not being believed that I was in labour because I sounded too calm was definitely a trigger. And being on pethidine was a trigger because being touched by people in a drugged state felt scary as I no longer felt I had any control.'

We must always be ready to have a conversation with a survivor in labour to reassure her and remind her that she is having a baby and that she is safe, to let her know that everything is normal and that this is not the abuse situation that she was once in. It is really important for a survivor to understand that something that has happened to her in the current situation has triggered memories and flashbacks from her past abuse.

Summary

- Avoid using language that can be triggers for survivors and always think about your choice of words and tone of voice.
- Become aware of behaviour that seems unusual, when women seem to be having flashbacks and be somewhere else.
- VEs are especially difficult for survivors so respect when women decline these. There are other ways of assessing labour progress.
- Always introduce yourself and explain in detail what it is that you are going to do, how long it will take and why you are doing it. Let the woman know that she has the option of saying 'no'.
- Touching of any kind always requires approval before it happens.

Identifiable behaviours in labour and birth

Labour and birth is a time when so much harm and trauma can be done to women by the people around them who they believe are there to care for them and show them kindness, compassion and dignity. Studies show us that regardless of the length of labour, the way the baby was born, the pain endured – nothing matters more than the way the women were treated by their caregivers. Feeling well cared for by nurses, midwives and doctors meant positive and satisfying experiences for women while feelings of being out of control as well as receiving disrespectful care from the medical professionals left women traumatised and with negative memories of their baby's birth (Simkin and Klaus 2004).

Simkin and Klaus write that, from published studies as well as their own experience in counselling sexual abuse survivors, they have learnt that survivors with unresolved abuse issues are more likely to feel poorly treated and misunderstood by their caregivers and experience complications in labour compared to women with no history of abuse (Simkin and Klaus 2004). In reality, this means that a large proportion of already traumatised women stand to become re-traumatised as well as experience complications during the birth of their baby as a direct result of the treatment they receive from the staff working at the time of their baby's birth.

There are a number of challenges for survivors in relation to labour and birth and they can be defined as being either intrinsic or extrinsic challenges. Intrinsic challenges are those things that the woman feels she has no control over and may feel very unpredictable to her, such as when labour will start, how long it will go on for and how painful it will be and concerns around how she will cope and manage it all. Extrinsic challenges are all of the procedures and routine care that happen in hospitals such as the hospital environment with bleeping machines and equipment and different medication and drugs; invasive procedures such as breaking the waters, putting cannulas in, VEs and taking blood samples and episiotomies. Survivors might worry about what type of equipment will be attached to them, such as blood pressure cuffs, continuous monitoring, and tubes and wires, such as epidurals and catheters. Will it be necessary to use instruments such as forceps and ventouse cups or will they need to have major stomach surgery? It can be a great worry just to meet with hospital staff, who to the survivor is usually a stranger, dressed in uniform and at times wearing a mouth guard.

Strong desire to be in control

Ultimately, sexual abuse of any kind is all about someone having power and control over someone who is or feels unable to defend themselves against it. It is often the case in CSA survivors that the abuser was also someone that the abused had to depend on in some way and someone that they should have been able to trust and rely on.

When it comes to childbirth, we can look at the aspects of being in control from three different angles: being in control of what is done to the woman by staff as well as her own birth partners; being in control of what her body is doing; and being in control of her own behaviours and responses to the sensations of labour (Simkin and Klaus 2004). Anything that happens in labour that feels like a caregiver has authority over the woman has the potential to leave a survivor traumatised again. It is paramount that the woman is fully involved and consulted in every single decision that is suggested during labour and birth. Any interaction with care providers where a survivor feels that trust and compliance is expected could be a reminder of her perpetrator.

It could be a major issue for survivors to lose control over their body as well as losing control of the contractions. The needs of the baby might become more important than the needs of the woman, making her feel like the baby is controlling her. It's not unusual for survivors to associate a lack of control with being abused.

If women are able to build positive and trusting relationships with their caregivers, who are also going to be there during labour and birth, the process can become a healing experience. For women to be able to feel safe, it is important that they are not triggered in any way that brings back memories of the abuse. If this happens, the care provided could be experienced as the re-enactment of past abuse (Montgomery 2013).

This strong need to stay in control might present itself differently from woman to woman and if the caregivers can recognise this behaviour for what it really is and respond to it from a trauma-informed directive, much healing and growth can be done. Survivors might either become aggressive, fighting and arguing with the staff, refusing to co-operate with anything or the opposite, become submissive and quiet, with overdependence on their partner and/ or caregivers, not wanting them to leave or worrying about being abandoned by them.

It might be worth marking a difference between 'losing control' and 'giving up control', both for the women themselves as well as those that care for them. The cocktail of hormones that the body is producing during a physiological birth might be something that women surrender to, as long as they are in a safe and trusting environment. It's a different thing if the way they are treated makes them feel as though their autonomy and decision-making is taken away. Women need to feel that they were given all the information that they needed when faced with a situation which they had hoped to avoid, for example an assisted or caesarean birth.

Dissociation

If a survivor has learnt to take herself away from a painful and threatening situation, it is possible that she will do the same if labour and birth become traumatic. As discussed above, she might seem like she's not present any more; perhaps she's unable to hear what is being said to hear and is not responding to questions. Dissociation is normally a survival technique to enable the person to cope with what is happening to them.

Sue talks about her memory of the birth of her first baby:

'The labour and birth seem to have been wiped from my memory. The only clear memories that I have are of a man (the husband of another woman) walking into the delivery room where I was on my own, with my legs in stirrups, waiting to be stitched.'

Some survivors find that dissociating is a way of coping with what is happening to them during labour and birth. Ebony had an emergency caesarean birth and this is how she describes it:

'I became very dissociated due to the shock and trauma (which was also my response to the abuse). Being numb and paralysed for the caesarean birth was not a good experience but was necessary. I was very uncomfortable at being handled by so many people though they were kind.'

As a caregiver with a woman who seems to have 'checked out', we need to pay extra attention to her. It is important to try and remain in eye-to-eye contact with her and keep talking to her, using her name, to make sure she can become present again.

It's important not to assume that a woman is coping well simply because she appears quiet and withdrawn. Sylvia explains:

'Women need to understand what is happening to them, at all times. A quiet, compliant woman is possibly suffering extreme distress.'

Request for female caregivers

Survivors often have a very strong desire to avoid caregivers of a certain sex, usually male caregivers; however, sometimes it could be female caregivers. It all depends on who their abuser was and who they feel they can trust and depend on the most.

Whilst a woman in a hospital can't demand to only have female caregivers, she has got the right to deny care from anyone that she doesn't want to care for her. This can, of course, become a problem if there is a medical emergency. Leila is still confused about what she experienced during labour which was also a huge trigger for her:

'It was only a few months afterwards that I felt that it had actually affected me and did wonder if it was related. I didn't think I would care, but he was so awful and in my mind unnecessarily grumpy and rough. I think for any future pregnancies I would now document that I am a survivor of abuse and to refuse VEs by any male caregiver. I don't know how in reality this would be though? What if there was only one consultant working and it was a male? Or would they just let a midwife do the examination?'

It seems that Leila suggests that any pre-conditioned ideas that a survivor has could have the potential to taint an experience with a male caregiver:

'The consultant came in to see me, who was male, he didn't have the nicest bedside manner and I felt at the time he was very rough when doing a VE. By this point I was so off my head

that I wasn't really thinking at all. I asked for an in-labour caesarean because I knew my body or baby would not react well to the Syntocinon and it would end up in an EMCS [Emergency Caesarean]. He left me for I don't know how long and came back to examine me again before taking me to theatre. Again, I felt it was unnecessarily rough. Actually I say I felt that. I didn't really at the time. It was awful but I didn't really think or process it.'

I believe that women need to be informed that they can decline any treatment as part of the consultation that should take place when consent is sought. If a woman asks for female caregivers and it is not for religious reasons, this should be taken seriously and potentially seen as a sign of that woman being a survivor of abuse.

Postdate pregnancies and dysfunctional labour

It's not unusual for survivors to have postdate pregnancies, to experience dysfunctional labour, leading to augmentation and even caesarean births. This could partly be down to the need to stay in control but also a belief that the body of a survivor is damaged and unable to start labour and progress until the baby is born. The survivor might also worry about becoming a mum so could be subconsciously stalling or halting her own progress (Erickson 1976).

We understand that any worry or stress produces hormones that inhibit the release of labour hormones and during the active phase of labour, when things might start to feel overwhelming or like the survivor can't cope and is losing control, she might start to release these hormones. It might be the case that she is keeping her labour at a level that she feels in control of and it might take her slightly longer to feel safe enough to let go into the process.

Invasive procedures for most women are worrying and scary but for a survivor, anything that is going to penetrate their body or cause damage may cause extreme fear. This includes a heightened fear of needles and IVs so any expressed concerns about this should be a potential red flag that you might be working with a survivor.

Anything that is going to penetrate any part of the body might be associated with being raped or abused again. Shanay talks about her experience of an induction as a survivor:

'I was induced. This meant fingers up my vagina, sweeps, and insertions of other things up there. I found all of that absolutely horrendous. I not only cried from the pain, but I felt invaded over and over again. Each time, I was reminded of my perpetrators. I knew they said there was no other way to kick-start the labour. It didn't change the trauma though.'

When I read this I wonder if Shanay did give informed consent to the induction: did she know that she could have declined? It breaks my heart when I read how a woman, on what should be one of the best days of her life, is being subjected to what in her eyes is abuse.

Leila planned for a home birth to stay away from the hospital environment but transferred as labour was not progressing according to the guidelines.

'I wanted a home birth, but didn't realise at the time that once the midwife was there you were kind of on a ticking clock. I had refused VEs but the midwife kept on and on saying that they had no idea where I was at, they couldn't have a baseline to see if I was progressing, etc. So reluctantly I agreed to one. It was kind of a cascade of stuff after that...not progressing well enough for their liking – then the suggestion of ARM, which I didn't really want to do at first but then felt like I kind of should or had to in order to try and avoid a transfer. The ARM was hideous and felt like the worst decision I had ever made...they couldn't break my waters and took several attempts, in the meantime I was having intense contractions and was having to stay in place whilst they kept trying.'

The coercion and constant requests to proceed with something that a survivor keeps saying 'no' to is, in itself, disrespecting her wishes and potentially leads to further interventions and traumatisation. I believe care providers need to take a step back and assess the whole situation and not simply focus on what they feel needs to be done. It can be documented in the notes that the woman declined an examination.

Other indicators

Survivors have a strong desire to stay in control and this means that it's not unusual for trauma survivors, not just from sexual abuse and violence, to have long and detailed birth plans. The birth plans often detail all the things that they don't want to be done to them and for many midwives and obstetricians, it can feel rather overwhelming to have this handed to them. A very detailed birth plan could be an indication that this woman has suffered some kind of trauma in the past and it might be a good idea to ask her about this. For example, you could ask, 'You have some very strong views on how you would like your birth to unfold, would you mind sharing with me if there are any specific reasons for this so that I can support you better?' At the end of the day, women's 'birth plans' are in reality a care plan of how they want to be treated, or not be treated, by their care providers.

From my own observations, survivors sometimes vomit more than other women in labour and appear to experience excessive pain and tension. They might appear hyper vigilant and panicky, fearful and suspicious of everyone and everything in the hospital. Often pain medication is quickly offered to women who appear to be in excessive pain, despite what might have been stated in a birth plan. Gita found it disappointing not to have other options presented to her but was also overwhelmed by the number of hospital staff present in the room:

'I really didn't want an epidural. Even when it was being set up and administered. I said to my husband I wanted everyone to go away and leave me alone but he didn't feel he had the voice to action this. A large number of hospital staff can feel really intimidating. Even with what professionals might consider to be in someone else's best interests, being neutral in offers of support seems really important to me.'

Cara explains how she opted for an epidural which, in the end, was the most triggering moment during the birth of her first child:

'I had an epidural that didn't work effectively and I was told I would have a Syntocinon drip that I definitely declined, but was given anyway. I begged my mum to let me die as the pain was so horrific and the lack of control scared me. This was the point which I still reflect on now as being the worst part.'

It makes total sense to assume that if a survivor cannot feel pain that it will be a more positive experience but we know from studies that it's not usually the pain that traumatises women; it's the way they are treated by the people around them.

Survivors are also more likely to feel upset about bodily fluids on their clothes, bedding or anywhere near them. They could be quite focused on cleanliness and worried about any germs or dirt in their birthing space.

They might also feel very worried about being naked or exposed to the caregivers that might be wandering in and out of the room. For others, it is impossible to be lying on their backs for labour and birth and the position the bed is in might be important. As mentioned, many survivors will feel vulnerable and exposed if their back is against the door so that they cannot see who is coming and going.

If you as a care provider notice scars from any self-harm on the woman you are supporting, this could be another marker that you are working with a survivor. In a longitudinal study, it was discovered that survivors of sexual abuse were four times more likely to self-harm (Noll *et al.* 2003).

Second stage of labour

Second stage of labour can often be a challenge to survivors as the feeling of the baby inside the vagina can bring back body memories of the abuse. The sensations during this stage of labour, the stretching and the worry about damage to the perineum can make women hold back. Just like many women worry about bowel movements during the birth, so do survivors, which is another thing that might prevent them from pushing their baby out. In some cases, a survivor might even see the baby as someone that is hurting her. She might also be feeling reluctant to become a parent.

Simkin and Klaus (2004) write about how important it is at this stage to reassure a survivor that she is pushing the pain out with the baby and to view the baby as a soldier in arms, ridding her of the pain. It can also help to let the woman sit on the toilet for a while, making the sensations be associated with bowel movements rather than with the abuse. It can help the woman relax her perineum and will help her to tune in to the bearing down sensations usually experienced in this stage of labour.

Supporting survivors during labour and birth

- Ensure the woman feels that she is part of the process, involved in all discussions and an equal partner in all decision-making.
- Make her feel that there are no power differences in the room by ensuring you communicate on the same level as her and use her name.
- Never touch or do anything to her without first asking permission and making sure you have given her all the information she will need.
- Listen – with your ears, with your heart, with your gut feeling. Focus on how you can make this a positive experience for this woman.
- Ask what you can do to support and help the woman in labour.
- Always knock on the door before entering and always introduce yourself.
- Respect the woman's wishes – if she declines treatment after you have given her all the information according to your professional guidelines, document this in the medical notes.
- Ensure that routines, procedures and guidelines don't become more important than your human interaction with the woman.

- Perceived demands of the institution should never take precedence over a woman's personal needs.

Nine clinical challenges and possible solutions – by Penny Simkin and Phyllis Klaus

In the book *When Survivors Give Birth* by Simkin and Klaus (2004), they include a specific list of clinical challenges in labour for survivors along with possible solutions. I've been given their kind permission to share this with you in this book.

1. Non-progressing contractions
Possible psychological causes
- Reluctance to enter the process that results in parenthood.
- Recognition that she is out of control over her body.
- Self-fulfilling prophecy: her body won't do this correctly because it is damaged, defective.

Possible solutions
- Talk it over. Why do you think it is taking so long to get into labour?
- Help her shift control from her body to her conscious responses to her contractions, which she can control.
- Reassurance that pre-labour often takes a long time, while the cervix ripens, effaces, and moves forward.
- Patience, nourishment, help with sleep (bath, massage, sleeping medications).

2. Resistance to or inability to tolerate vaginal exams, blood draws, IVs, catheters, etc.
Possible psychological causes
- Association with rape or genital pain, especially if done by same gender as her perpetrator.
- Phobia over blood.
- Invasion of body boundaries may represent a metaphor for rape, defencelessness, etc.
- Fear of having genitals exposed, visible to strangers.

Possible solutions

- Let her know she can decline (doulas). Do as few of these procedures as possible and tell her that (midwife/doctor).
- Ideally, should have been discovered before labour and noted prominently on her notes.
- ALWAYS get the woman's permission.
- Proceed slowly, step by step, regulated by the woman.
- Have a trusted, kind, familiar person with her – a doula!
- Respect her modesty as much as possible.

3. Strong preferences for one care provider or gender of care provider

Possible psychological causes

- Distrust of authority figures of that gender (associated with gender of perpetrator).
- Client may believe other women are, like her or like her mother, weak, incompetent, untrustworthy or evil.

Possible solutions

- Validate her need and try very hard to honour this need (and, if impossible, tell her that you tried).
- Ideally, should have been discovered ahead of time.
- If possible, arrange for person of client's desired gender to do vaginal exams and other invasive procedures.
- Use active listening; try not to take it personally (midwives/doctors/medical staff).

4. Labour progress stalls in active phase

Possible psychological causes

- Labour pain is reaching a point where she can no longer remain in control. Deep fear of pain behaviours (screaming, thrashing and panicking) associated with being helpless and out of control during abuse. She keeps the labour at a level where she can remain in control.
- Deep fear of vaginal birth, preference for a caesarean for failure to progress.
- Fear leads to increased production of stress hormones (catecholamine), known to slow labour.

Possible solutions
- Talk it over: why do you think your progress has stalled?
- Pain medications or an epidural may diminish the output of catecholamines, and enable further interventions, such as oxytocin or second-stage interventions.

5. Struggling during administration of epidural, even though she requested it
- Possible psychological causes
- Anaesthesia placed by unseen person at her back may remind her of abuse from behind at night.
- Reminders to lie still and it will be over sooner, may be what she heard before.
- If birth partner is asked to leave for the procedures, it magnifies her helplessness.

Possible solutions
- Speak to her face to face before beginning procedure.
- Describe every step.
- Ask her for feedback.
- Have her partner or doula at her face and the nurse offering encouragement and praise.
- If necessary, speak firmly and confidently. No coaxing or sweet-talking.

6. Woman appears out-of-touch, in a trance, and it is difficult or impossible to speak with her (dissociation, blanking out)
Possible psychological causes
- This may be a survival technique, used since childhood to leave during pain or terror.
- Dissociation blocks not only the experience, but any memory of it as well.

Possible solutions
- If possible, find out ahead of time if she sometimes dissociates, and how she feels about it for labour.
- If she doesn't want to dissociate, her partner, doula, midwife or caregiver should maintain eye contact, keep talking to her and ask her to respond by words and actions. Keep her in the present.

7. Delay or failure in descent in second stage
Possible psychological causes
- Fear of vaginal birth: the pain, stretching, possible tearing, episiotomy.
- Perception of the baby as perpetrator, hurting and damaging her.
- Reluctance to become a parent.
- Holding back tension in perineum.
- Fear of exposure or expelling faeces.

Possible solutions
- Reassurance.
- Associate birth more with bowel movement than rape.
- Remind her that the pain is coming out of her body; the baby is her ally in getting rid of the pain.
- Cover her vaginal outlet and perineum with a hot compress.
- Ask her why she thinks the baby is not coming.
- Episiotomy, vacuum extractor, forceps (will not solve underlying emotional reasons).

8. Lack of interest in the newborn; wants father or others to hold baby; resists attempts by staff to give baby to mother
Possible psychological causes
- Perception of the baby as perpetrator.
- Dissociation during birth may delay bonding.
- Traumatic birth may over-ride thoughts for baby.
- Abuse in childhood may have left the woman with little instinct of mothering.

Possible solutions
- Allow expressions of anger, lack of confidence, dislike toward the baby.
- Encourage a more positive family member to be with the baby.
- Don't rush contact between mother and baby. Give the mother time to recognise that labour is over, to come back. Most abuse survivors do take in the baby.
- Model ways to hold the child; encourage positive gestures by the mother; point out how the baby responds to her; show her infant cues.
- Make sure the mother has resources and follow-up after leaving hospital.

9. Reluctance or inability to breastfeed

Possible psychological causes

- Flashbacks to abuse brought on by the baby having access to breasts, sucking and hurting them.
- Perception of the baby as perpetrator, manipulative, wilful, hurtful, selfish.
- Modesty issues around exposure of breasts.

Possible solutions

- Recognise that sometimes abuse survivors cannot breastfeed. Follow their lead.
- Pumping and feeding by bottle may be acceptable as an alternative.
- Help mother recognise that a young baby cannot manipulate or deliberately hurt her. Help her frame her perceptions.
- Refrain from touching the woman's breasts; allow privacy. Teach latch techniques without making her expose her breast. Let her try in private.

Chapter 3

Things to Consider

Consent and human rights

There are very clear laws in the UK around informed consent and human rights in relation to maternity care. All UK public bodies are bound by the law and must provide maternity care that is respectful of women's dignity, autonomy and equality. Just like everyone is entitled to make decisions about their own body, so are pregnant women and no one can give any kind of medical treatment to a woman without her agreeing to it. Consent must be obtained before any treatment can be carried out and the same goes for any examination or investigation. A woman might give consent to a certain procedure at one time but that doesn't mean that consent doesn't need to be given for that procedure again. It's also the woman's right to withdraw consent, that is, ask a medical professional to stop what they're doing immediately.

It's very clear legally what 'consent' actually means and it involves a person genuinely agreeing to receive the treatment that is being offered. For a woman in labour to give personal consent, she must be well-enough informed about the proposed treatment and should not have been put under undue influence, pressured or bullied into receiving the treatment by healthcare professionals or a family member.

Sue felt that during the birth of her first baby, there was no one there listening to her. She was 17 at the time and had suffered abuse at the hands of her father from an early age:

'I never felt that I was able to give any kind of consent for anything that happened to me. It was as though the whole

experience was taken out of my hands. I think being so young I was treated as a child and my care providers didn't respect my decisions. It felt that I was just caught up in a process and nobody was sufficiently experienced enough to pick up the signs of my distress. By this I mean my dissociation. As I continue to understand what happened to me, I realise now that I needed to do this. The impact that this has had on me is huge.'

I believe it is vitally important for all birth workers to remember that for every woman having a baby it is a new and fresh experience. You might have seen this many times before and become desensitised from the intervention or procedure but for the woman it's all new. When I asked Sue if she had any 'top tips' for care providers; her answer was:

'My top tip for care providers would be to never assume what you are about to say or do to a woman is something that they are comfortable with. The language used. The examinations. Women need to be fully informed at all stages whether survivors or not about what is going to happen to them.'

No healthcare professional should unduly influence a woman to accept their advice and the information about the treatment must include the risk of the procedure to the woman and her unborn child, other alternatives and the risk of doing nothing. The healthcare professional can recommend a particular clinical opinion; however, if you, as a healthcare professional, resort to physical restraint, threaten to withdraw care, keep repeating unwanted discussions of risk, put a deadline on when the decision must be made or put pressure on other family members to put pressure on the woman, you could be breaking the law. All of these behaviours could be seen as undue influence and in breach of UK laws.

Georgia explained how the way her midwife supported her helped:

'I think it's important for care providers to be cautious of physical touch. And wording. Also ask for consent. Also explain

before touching and ask if that is OK. My midwife did that and it helped a lot.'

It has been known in the past that health professionals will use the threat of reporting women to social services if they don't accept a recommended treatment. This kind of intimidating, bullying or coercing is also classified as undue influence and should simply not be happening. It is every woman's human right to decline treatment, for any reasons, rational or irrational, or for no reason at all. This is the case even if it means the woman losing her own life.

The way consent is obtained in maternity care is often outside of guidelines and I have seen this on many occasions when supporting clients as a doula. It's often assumed that women will comply with what the clinical guidelines say rather than deal with all the risks and alternatives being discussed. I often hear healthcare providers use statements such as: 'We're now going to [insert procedure], is that OK?' or 'We need to [insert procedure], are you OK with that?' Most women assume that they have to do what is being suggested and go along with the procedure, not having been given all the information so an informed choice could be made. Survivors are especially vulnerable when it comes to giving consent as once consent has been given, they might be unable to withdraw consent during the procedure. During the assault they experienced in the past, they might have responded by going into a freeze state, which might happen again during any procedure to which they first consented (as discussed above). It might also be the case that they dissociate if the procedure is triggering. Gita explains how she was unable to tell her care provider to stop the VE that she didn't feel she had consented to in the first place:

'Not saying "don't do that to me" because my voice was frozen was considered as me giving consent for sexual assault to the perpetrator. It felt the same in the birthing room...not having my voice at that moment in time as it froze meant that I wasn't giving consent.'

For a woman to give informed consent she needs to have all the information about the risks of each option. Inductions of labour are often advised by medical professionals and the risks of not taking that medical advice are often clearly pointed out whilst, in my experience, the risks of the induction are rarely explained. Georgia felt, in hindsight, that she was not given enough information about her induction, nor was she given alternatives.

> *'I felt as though I did not give informed consent during my labour and birth. I had to be induced 24 hours after a high water leakage but it very much was not given to me as an option but an order. And with that came the IV, the heart monitors and that felt very restricting. It felt like it took my power away.'*

Article 8 of the European Convention on Human Rights guarantees the right to private life, which in principle means a woman must always give her informed consent before anything is done to her.

It's very simple: women can make choices about their own maternity care and healthcare professionals must respect those choices, even if they don't agree with them. There are no laws around maternity care that women have to adhere to. Women do not have to tell anyone that they are pregnant; they don't have to attend antenatal appointments or scans or have any tests done in pregnancy. A woman does not have to have medically trained support present when she gives birth and can birth wherever she wants with whomever she chooses, as long as that person does not perform any kind of midwifery functions. The only legal requirement is that the birth of the child must be registered at the local register office within a specific time frame, depending on where in the UK you live. All births in England, Wales and Northern Ireland must be registered within 42 days of the child being born and, in Scotland, births must be registered within 21 days.

A wonderful organisation which deals with human rights in maternity is Birthrights, which has a number of downloadable fact sheets and also runs workshops for healthcare professionals.

Communication

Communication can be seen as a two-way system in which someone talks and the other party listens. We are usually aware of the fact that everyone hears what is being said differently, depending on their culture, life experience and current state of mind. A group of 20 people will potentially all interpret and process any information in their own unique way. This means they will also make up their own version of what is 'true' and create a memory of what was said, based on any previous knowledge and experiences that are similar to the information they received.

If we experience something that evokes an emotional response, we usually try to make sense of the situation and often we will do this by making up a 'story' based on what we already know. This means that a lot of the birth stories women are told by other women often don't make sense and are often factually incorrect. What we hear is how this woman experienced the birth of her baby and, after telling it many times, having solutions and fixes added by those around her, she has created a story which makes sense to her and fills in all the gaps. I'm not suggesting that women are lying or making things up, what I am saying is that what we're hearing is how she experienced her birth and how she has since made sense of it. It is not necessarily exactly what happened; instead, it is her interpretation of it. It doesn't really matter what the caregivers around her feel happened or how they interpreted the situation. If a woman feels that she was unkindly treated and feels traumatised after her experience then that is the memory that she is left with and we have failed her.

When we communicate with women, whether they are survivors or not, we need to be very sensitive with the words we use, the way we put our information across, and the tone of voice in which we communicate. Pregnant women are more likely to be extremely sensitive to anything that might sound judgemental or harsh, or comes across as criticism. Especially if they are survivors as they might already feel defensive but also fearful of what is going to happen to them during their time at the hospital or clinic.

The words we use when communicating, especially during pregnancy and birth, have a huge impact on women, the way they feel about their bodies and their ability to give birth. Being mindful of the way we communicate is such a simple thing, and can have such a huge impact.

My children used to sing a song at assembly when they were at primary school, and some of the words were: 'Your tongue's a tiny part of your body, but such enormous harm can be done by it. Every time you open your mouth, you've got to think before you speak.' I think the text is wonderful, and simply explains how careful we should be with the words we use.

In the antenatal period

When women are told that they have developed a pregnancy-related problem, the information they are given is often confusing for them, and may be delivered in a manner that can leave them stressed and upset. In my experience, the perceived risk of something going wrong is often not very clearly expressed, and data and statistics are often misunderstood by the pregnant woman. Instead of offering real numbers to compare, statistics are often communicated as 'double the chance' or 'increased risks'. If something doubles from something that was small in the first place, there is still more of a chance that everything will still be fine.

Women need to have clear and simple information so that they understand the situation rather than the emotional blackmail that sometimes takes place. If the risk factor is 1 in 200, it might be easier for a woman to understand if it is also presented as a 0.5 per cent risk or, even better, a 99.5 per cent chance of it not happening. To make a sweeping statement that there is an increased risk of having a baby that is unwell or stillborn naturally frightens the woman and she may be unable to think rationally about how to proceed.

Most of the time, there is also no mention of the risks associated with medical interventions, such as the increased risks in a caesarean birth after a medically induced induction of labour (Vardo *et al.*

2011). Or that clinical guidelines, such as continuous foetal monitoring during labour for women with low-risk pregnancies, increase the chances of a caesarean birth by 20 per cent – with no known evidence that there are any benefits for doing this (Devane *et al.* 2017).

When care providers are simply following a set of written guidelines without engaging with the pregnant woman on an emotional level, much damage can be done. Of course, they need to convey what they need to, but they should always remember what the potential impact could be on their patient. Women listen with their hearts when they are pregnant, so only need to hear what is going to be helpful to them and relevant at the time. Information should, of course, not be kept from a pregnant woman, but the way it is presented and communicated should be a priority. It should be left to the woman to make up her own mind and choose what she feels is right for her.

In labour

Words can mean so many different things to different people, and having the sensitivity to consider how we say things could prevent someone from suffering unnecessarily or re-living a trauma. We all have words that trigger reactions in us in one way or another, and different words can be triggers to different people.

Simkin and Klaus, in their book *When Survivors Give Birth* (2004), explain that especially during times of stress, the words and actions of a caregiver can elicit unexpected behaviours in childhood abuse survivors.

They list the following phrases, usually said to be helpful but which could potentially be the same words that are used by an abuser:

- 'Open your legs.'
- 'Relax your bottom.'
- 'This will hurt only a little.'
- 'Relax, and it won't hurt so much.' (Simkin and Klaus 2004)

Paula has really strong feelings when it comes to language, in particular care providers using 'good girl' when referring to the women they look after. She says:

'Absolutely under no circumstances say things like "good girl" as this can have a psychological impact of transporting that woman back to a time of childhood abuse where the abuser may have used exactly those words. More generally speaking, calling a full-grown woman "girl" is also psychologically belittling and reinforces feelings of powerlessness and not feeling able to take full responsibility.'

There are also many disempowering phrases used about women's bodies that when you actually take a look, it becomes so obvious how unhelpful or judgemental most of these are.

Words that disempower and criticise the woman's body:

- caesarean section – we talk about people with mental illness being 'sectioned'
- delivery/delivered – as many people have said before, pizzas are delivered, grapefruit is sectioned and babies are birthed!
- pain relief – it sounds as though the pain is a bad thing and needs to be taken away
- contractions – something is being pulled together; it sounds painful
- failure to progress – this implies it is the woman's fault that she is not progressing in labour
- lack of maternal effort – sounds as if the woman can't be bothered to birth her baby
- incompetent cervix – sounds as if the woman's body is failing
- lazy uterus – again, sounds as if the woman's body is failing.

Words to use instead:

- caesarean birth – refers to a baby being born, rather than a woman 'sectioned'; sounds more active and babies are always born

- birth/birthed – the woman always births her baby; no one delivers it
- pain management – sounds more positive, as if the pain can be managed
- surges/rushes – talks about the hormones surging, causing the uterus to work.

A woman's body very rarely 'fails' to give birth to her baby, but, in my experience, often she does not get the right support and is not giving birth in an environment in which she feels safe. Any phrases referring to the woman's body failing are better labelled as an 'unsupportive environment'.

Phrases and words randomly used when supporting a woman in labour and birth could bring back bad memories, or memories she has hidden away in the back of her mind. We are as we are for a reason and, at times, birth professionals and birth partners might be the target for a labouring woman's unexpressed feelings. However, the birthing woman needs empathy and compassion, not harsh words or punishment for not complying.

Gita talks about how communication was important to her experience:

'When care providers spoke to me with respect and dignity I felt a deep healing in my body, conversely when I felt violated and an examination was performed without my consent I felt my trust had been broken. I have a deep empathy with the busyness of a midwifery unit. I believe all midwives are working from a place of love and care, it's just that sometimes seeing a woman in labour as a unique individual rather than 'room X patient' can be challenging when working under pressure.'

In the postnatal period

As a doula, I have seen first-hand what well-meaning hospital staff, partners and family members say to women who have just had a baby.

A story I have heard many times is about a new mum in hospital who puts her baby on her bed without making sure she can't roll off, and is told off by a member of staff for not keeping her baby safe. Also, women are often given overwhelming and confusing information about breastfeeding. For many women, being told off when they have just started out as a mother can have a long-lasting effect on how they feel about themselves as a competent mother. It's a confusing time and, as a new mother finds her feet and her own ways of being a mum, she needs to be talked to with kindness and gentleness.

There are guidelines and recommendations for keeping a baby safe, but there is no reason why these can't be communicated in a caring manner. No new mother should be told off for doing the best she can with the information that she has at the time. Time and time again, women tell me how they can remember when someone said something mean to them during birth or in the postnatal period. It is difficult for new mums not to take to heart things that have been said to them when their bodies are aching, their lives have been turned upside down, and they are desperate for some nurturing and kindness.

If women expect to encounter people who are not going to say helpful things in the postnatal period, they can choose to ignore what is said to them. If women realised that they are the experts on how to look after their baby, they can choose what information they take on board and what to ignore, and trust their instincts.

Signposting

It always surprises me that medically trained care providers often feel unsure about signposting women who might need more support to independent birth workers, such as doulas. Many doulas are skilled in offering counselling services, trauma-healing techniques and other complementary therapies. To have this continuity of support can make a real difference to women, and in particular to survivors. Sylvia talks about how she believes having continuity of support would have made a difference to her:

'If I'd been able to build a relationship with someone during pregnancy I might have been able to disclose to her and if she had been able to care for me during labour, my experience might have been much better.'

Ellen had similar feelings about the external support she would have liked:

'I know there is a referral to prenatal psychologist but for us survivors many of us have been over this with a psychologist and just don't want to go there again. A counsellor that could discuss hypnobirthing with us, go over our rights with us (so we know we can say no) and maybe some CBT would be brilliant. Failing that, the NHS suggesting sessions with a doula that can do just that would be ground breaking for us.'

Shanay made the suggestion that it might be worth always having a trained counsellor or therapist to call on when someone with previous mental health issues is in labour. It may seem like rather a simple solution that the support some women need the most during childbirth is someone to talk to about what they are going through and what is perhaps coming to the surface. Shanay says:

'I wish that a counsellor/psychologist/psychotherapist had been on hand. I was in the hospital for four days. In that time, I wish a professional had been there to provide talk therapy through the process. Birth was not just a physical activity, it was as much mental. Doctors, anaesthetists, etc. were on hand. As someone who has had mental illness all my life, the biggest health concern was totally unsupported.'

It seems that we have some support in place for women who have mental health issues during pregnancy, although this is still very poor in most NHS trusts around the country. Hopefully, this will improve as further funding and plans for improvement are in place (NHS England 2019). Postnatally, we seem to have more understanding and GPs are able to support many new mothers suffering from depression. However, it seems to me absolutely absurd that we don't offer anything during labour, a chance for women to be able to talk about previous experiences, learn more about their options in an honest and objective way and have mental health specialists on call who specialise in maternity as well as trauma.

There is an excellent new therapy that is being shown to make a difference in treating PTSD called Eye Movement Desensitisation and Reprocessing (EMDR) (as mentioned in Chapter 2). In a very recent pilot study, an intense five-day treatment programme with EMDR as well as yoga reduced the symptoms of PTSD (Zepeda Méndez *et al.* 2018). Perhaps we should look into offering these kinds of therapies to survivors of sexual abuse and violence as well as signposting them to having a doula support them.

Vicarious traumatisation

As maternity workers, we might find ourselves in a position of listening to detailed and harrowing stories about traumatic experiences that the women we support have been through, for example a survivor's story of sexual abuse. As we tend to engage in an empathic way, the trauma can be transferred as we are exposed to the details. This is called vicarious traumatisation, also known as secondary traumatisation, secondary stress disorder or insidious trauma. So even if you were not an immediate witness of the trauma, you absorb and integrate the disturbing aspects of the incident and this may leave you traumatised.

The symptoms of vicarious traumatisation are of the same nature as those caused by being exposed to trauma directly as well as symptoms related to PTSD. The symptoms are similar but tend to be of a lesser nature. However, if you already have PTSD or if you're a survivor of abuse yourself, you could be more open to re-traumatisation.

I believe that many of the workers in the NHS are suffering with PTSD of some form and probably at different levels. There needs to be better support for our midwives and doctors so that they can work from a healthy place and not respond from a place of avoidance based on previous trauma.

It is important to monitor yourself and keep track of levels of burnout as well as compassion fatigue. When faced with difficult accounts told by women, it can be helpful to tell yourself that this is not your story and not your pain to hold on to. It is, of course, also important to take regular breaks, making sure all your basic needs are met and, if you need external help, you should seek support from appropriate services.

Even though we want to help others, it's also important to set boundaries not only for the women and families we work with but also with our places of employment. Ensure you get to attend training for your different roles so that you can feel confident and supported in what you do.

Top tips for supporting survivors

There needs to be more training for healthcare professionals about the impact of sexual abuse and sexual violence on childbearing women. There simply is not enough importance put on learning bedside manner, showing empathy and understanding, which are extremely important when supporting women who are pregnant and giving birth to their babies. This is true for all women but especially for women who are survivors. The care of women needs more focus as well as recognising the challenges and triggers that are unique for women who are survivors.

It's not just the care providers such as midwives, consultants and maternity care assistants who look after women during the childbearing years but also all hospital staff, such as receptionists, cleaners, product representatives, volunteers and catering staff. This includes, in the community, health visitors and GPs too. This is expressed by Shanay in my communications with her:

> 'There is no place for [that kind of] ignorance and insensitivity when you're dealing with women in their most vulnerable state.'

It is vitally important that a woman who is coming through the maternity system is kindly and respectfully treated by everyone that she comes in contact with.

Improve communication

To be listened to and understood was a major theme running through the feedback I had from my questionnaires when I asked for survivors to give me their top tips for care providers. Often the women I heard back from felt not only that they were not heard but also that their care providers did not connect with them or treat them like a person. Sylvia explains:

> 'Talk to me! Put me in control. Help me feel safe. Look me in the eye and connect with me. My over-riding memory of childbirth, both times, is feeling LONELY. Even the people who talked to me didn't actually CONNECT with me.'

Cara had similar feelings:

> 'You should have listened to me, realised this was not normal behaviour, even without knowing my past, my behaviour was that of someone terrified.'

Communication is not simply about using words; we know from studies that body language says more than words (Mehrabian 1972; Calero 2005).

Sharon had a simple suggestion on what would have improved the care that she had during her baby's birth. Her message to care providers is:

> 'To choose words carefully and remember even if mum is in deep labour to make sure she is spoken to and not about behind her back.'

Paula's suggestions and top tip for care providers make complete sense and I believe would have a huge impact for all women:

'Always assume that this woman may have been abused as a child or young woman, rather than assume they haven't. And understand that women who have been abused in the past may have self-esteem issues or lack confidence to say no to things.'

What most women want is to be seen as an individual who is experiencing something for the first time whilst those of us working in maternity care will have become accustomed to what happens on the wards. Holly expresses how she is still feeling after her birth experience:

'That woman is in a very vulnerable position, even though it is your everyday norm, it is an event in my life that I will never forget. Do you want that woman to remember your actions forever as I have? Believe them when they say that they are experiencing pain, everyone feels it differently and just because I am not acting how you would expect me to, that doesn't mean that my pain is not genuine.'

It's understandable that it can be frustrating working in a system which is pushed to its limits with little support and care for the staff but this should not be taken out on the most vulnerable, the women you provide care for.

Aggressive and bullying behaviour will never be a sensible route to take and will leave women with negative memories. I realise that sometimes it's done to bring focus so that women in labour will get the job done, so to speak; however, it can have the opposite impact. Esme's message for her care provider is:

'Not screaming at me: "I can't do this for you; you have to do it now!" It frightened me and made me feel like I was responsible for my baby being in danger.'

Ellen had some suggestions around what would be helpful for a survivor:

> *'Give space, not to feel like you are being watched. Observation from a distance is better. Don't repeatedly touch women to check baby's heart tone or feel the tummy for contractions. Don't repeatedly do vaginal examinations and ideally just once if really needed. Look for other signs of progression. No directed pushing unless really needed either. Same goes for telling a woman to stop pushing. It's such a trigger to be told to do something or not to do something. If it's really needed, please choose your words carefully so it doesn't feel like she has no choice.'*

Informed consent

As part of obtaining informed consent, we must learn how to communicate effectively, to give information in an objective way, ensuring women are given references to the research as well as being clear on the actual numbers when discussing risk and avoiding phrases such as 'high risk' or 'increased risk'.

Informed consent is often not practised and, instead, we get more of the paternalistic medical model, that is, the belief that only the doctor can and should make the decision around what care is needed, which takes the power and autonomy away from women. This is an outdated model and not what a woman-centred maternity system should look like. There needs to be more focus on ensuring that relevant guidelines, written for all maternity workers, are better understood and adhered to. They all have the same message. The Royal College of Obstetrics and Gynaecologists (RCOG) says clearly what should happen:

> To obtain informed consent the process of shared understanding and decision making between patient and clinician must be approached diligently and robustly. Before seeking a woman's consent for a test, treatment, intervention or operation, you should ensure that she is fully informed, understands the nature of the condition for which it

is being proposed, its prognosis, likely consequences and the risks of receiving no treatment, as well as any reasonable or accepted alternative treatments. Uncertainties that the woman may have about the management of the condition should be discussed. (Royal College of Obstetrics and Gynaecologists 2015)

These guidelines are similar for midwives and nurses and also in line with the latest UK law on informed consent. They make it very clear that a woman should be 'fully informed' of everything before anything is done to her. Although in a busy maternity unit time isn't always on the side of the staff working there, Georgia's top tip is as follows:

'My top tip for care providers would be to explain everything to the woman as though she knew absolutely nothing about the process. Explain to her every little detail so that she feels safe and knowledgeable. And after that, ask her for her consent to do anything, whether it is a blood test, an induction, a caesarean, feeling her stomach, anything.'

Gita suggests that if the caregivers know about previous abuse they should talk about it in a normal way and ask if any additional support or more information might be needed so that informed consent can be given. She asks caregivers:

'With or without knowledge, to be patient, to know informed consent isn't getting someone to agree with you.'

Ellen remembers what was most difficult during her births:

'Being in hospital and feeling like I couldn't say no. Some midwives and doctors are really bad at giving you every scare story, or telling you that you have no choice. Many will tell you that you are in danger or your child is in danger but never back this up. Scare tactics to get a woman to go with their way of thinking. Ask consent for everything. Even if it's just a urine sample say something like 'Would you mind giving me a urine

sample so I can check it?' instead of 'I need a urine sample now.'
Explain why you are doing something and if writing notes let
the woman read them or read it over with her afterwards, don't
hide anything.'

Touching

It is true that in normal life, we don't usually touch people we do not know and we ensure we apologise if we do accidentally. When it comes to maternity services and pregnant women, it seems that some of these socially accepted no-nos disappear. Anna, who is a survivor and doula, explains:

'I think healthcare professionals need to get their hands off women. I'm now a doula and I see midwives and obstetricians touch women all the time and women allow it or think it's normal. If you're a survivor touch can be hugely triggering, especially by a man. I saw one obstetrician once pat a woman's bare thigh as he reassured her that her baby would be OK as they were going to do a caesarean. In no other circumstance would a man do this or think this is OK so why is it OK in birth?'

There are a number of checks and measurements that caregivers might like to do during labour but sometimes women are not asked consent as these procedures are carried out automatically. Women often experience a stripping of their bodily autonomy as procedures are carried out without explanation or consent. It may appear as if women are making a big fuss over small things but it's the overall sense of having their power and identity taken away, not being heard and not given options. Ellen explains one of her greatest challenges during the birth of her baby:

'Not being asked if I wanted blood pressure done or bloods and just assuming that I would. I found them just assuming I would want my fundal height checked and the way some of them touched me to be really tough.'

I can imagine it becomes routine to carry out many of the checks that medical care providers are asked to do by the clinical guidelines in place. It can be assumed that women will understand that what you are doing is necessary and done because it will keep the woman and her baby safe. I understand that having to ask all the time feels strange as you get to know each other but there really is only one way to get consent and that is by asking. The way the questions should be formulated is so that the woman can answer 'yes' or 'no'. Asking for consent is not saying 'I need to listen in to your baby' but instead 'I would like to listen to your baby's heart tone; is that OK with you?' Touching women without asking first is guaranteed to be a trigger for survivors so make sure you do ask before touching any part of their body, with your hands or with equipment.

Chapter 4

Working with Survivors

The Postnatal Period

Becoming a mum

I don't believe any woman is ever ready for the enormous changes that having a baby brings. It's a time of major transformation and often feels like a complete identity crisis for most women. The lack of sleep, lack of time for oneself, the overwhelming feelings of having to look after another human being can throw a woman's life into turmoil. Even the women that were looking forward to becoming mothers will at some point question if they made the right decision. This time in a woman's life was coined by Dana Raphael as 'matresence', the transition into motherhood (1976), and recently brought to life by a TED talk by Dr Alexandra Sachs (2018). This definition is a way of normalising the period around childbirth by comparing it to the confusing and major changes that take place in adolescence. Many of the emotions that women go through in this period are to be expected, especially since, in our modern society, many of us have lost the 'village' that would have been there to support and help us through this phase of life.

For survivors, this period can also bring additional challenges and it can often be confusing for them to know if what they are feeling is something that is universal or if it's because of their abuse in the past.

Survivors won't experience all of the additional challenges but most will be able to identify with some or many of them.

Challenges for survivors postnatally

Since survivors might already have mental health issues, such as depression, and might already struggle with the daily challenges of life, the additional stresses from caring for a baby could lead to postnatal mental health issues, such as anxiety, PTSS, PTSD or even a psychosis. They might physically be unwell and their recovery time might take longer. Often, relationships might suffer, especially with their partners and parents, even more so, of course, if one of the parents was the abuser. There can be a real struggle between keeping the children safe and sadness around denying them access to their grandparents. Georgia explains how some of her struggles played out after the birth of her baby:

'I had terrible anxiety postpartum. It has also been extremely difficult for me to be intimate with my husband since giving birth. Still 14 months later. By intimate I mean everything from hugging to sex. I find even cuddling or kissing really hard. It is hard to surrender. I would say those two things, anxiety and intimacy, have been the hardest.'

Survivors often grow up with a negative self-image and this can lead to setting extremely high standards for themselves so they can be at risk of becoming perfectionists. The strong desire to be a 'perfect mum' and ensure that no one can criticise them for the way they are bringing up their baby can become overwhelming eventually. If a family member was the abuser, the realisation that someone that you should be able to love and trust subjected you to so much hurt often also comes to the surface and the worry that this could happen to the survivor's children can be crippling. It can mean that the survivor becomes unable to ask anyone for help or even allow anyone else to care for her children, even her partner. Sue talks about this:

'I breastfed all of my children. I was not going to have anyone tell me that I wasn't doing my best. Again it was probably another step in the need for me to have complete care for them. Everything becomes so mixed up. The strong desire to be the perfect mum. The absolutely crippling anxiety and pain that comes with the realisation that somebody can commit such evil acts on a child. Everything came crashing down when my first child was two. I knew that I had to tell someone. I had an amazing health visitor. I remember just before she was coming round for a visit I was rushing round making sure everything was perfect. House tidy, baby clean, nothing out of place. I knew that I couldn't continue like this so it all came out in that visit. It was like a door had been unlocked.'

It's not unusual for survivors to become overly protective of their children as they can identify with the helplessness and vulnerability of their baby and start to worry about all possible potential dangers in the future. Other survivors recognise the stigma around sexual abuse and worry about how to be a 'good' parent; a survivor might feel anxious about molesting her baby or causing the baby pain. Paula describes these difficult feelings:

'If your boundaries were breached – you have to learn them anew and put them in place with your own child. I remember being a bit terrified of changing my child's nappy, of even touching his genitals at all, and feeling so so anxious not to repeat the cycle of abuse or make mistakes with boundaries – where can you go to learn this stuff? It's a skill like any other, but so many parents who were abused themselves must go through these feelings without anywhere to turn. I had to figure it out all on my own, bottling it all up then crying in the arms of my husband. I felt ashamed, I felt stigma, I worried that if I talked about being abused and asked questions about how to be a good healthy parent, that it might be marked against my name as a reason for concern – again, more stigma.'

Melanie shared her feelings around this:

> *'I left care at 16, living alone in a flat, supporting myself and trying to find my own way through life was the only way, nobody had my back, nobody guided me, nobody wanted to hear me. Alone, damaged and unsupported. Late one night I watched a documentary about child abuse and it contained a set of statistics that stated a high percentage of abused children in turn become abusers themselves. My world at this very moment fell apart; this is what I would be? I might as well end my life, what life was I to have anyway?'*

Sue talks about the overwhelming feelings she had about protecting her baby:

> *'Once my baby was born I became like a lion with her cub. I didn't want anyone touching her and I remember feeling like I would never be able to sleep again. Such was my fear of letting her out of my sight. This continued into the postnatal period. This in hindsight was going to be the beginning of my recovery.'*

Other challenges faced by survivors are issues around breastfeeding and it is important for women to separate the act of feeding a baby from any sexual associations around the breasts. A survivor could be triggered by the baby on the breast and it could even feel like incest or that she's forcing the baby on the breast. It's especially important when supporting women in the postnatal period with feeding issues that consent is given before any part of the woman's body is touched. Grabbing a woman's breast and shoving it into the baby's mouth will not be helpful to anyone, especially not to survivors. As mentioned earlier, if having the baby suckling on the breast is a big trigger for the woman, expressing and feeding breast milk in a bottle could be a solution but only if this is an acceptable option for the woman.

It's during times like this that banging on about how 'breast is best' could do a lot of harm rather than work as motivation. All women need to be well supported with breastfeeding, without any pressure about one way being best whilst another is bad.

Ellen speaks about feeding her babies:

'I bottle fed all my babies. I had real issues feeding the first three as I didn't produce milk. I did get some milk with my fourth but I couldn't bring myself to feed him. I did try with my fifth but I found it too tough to feed him. I managed nine days when my daughter left NICU [newborn intensive care unit] with combination feeding but again I found it really tough to feed her. I wanted nothing more than to feed her but something had blocked in me emotionally and I found it so tough and would get very emotional. For me it wasn't worth it so I switched to formula only. I believe it might have helped if I'd had better breastfeeding support without having to wait days to be seen to talk about it. These appointments need to be long enough so the woman can take her time and not feel rushed.'

In the end, there is a red thread running through this whole book and it keeps coming back to listening. All survivors and all women in the childbearing years really want is for someone to listen to what they want to do and listen to what they are telling you.

Esme found that after telling staff at the hospital in a postnatal meeting about her abuse that she felt as though she had been put under surveillance but also was not being supported with her feeding choices:

'I didn't like health visitors visiting me all the time. I felt like I was being checked up on. Or trying to be controlled. I felt forced to try bottle feeding when I was battling through breast feeding.'

Not surprisingly, what will make the biggest difference in the postnatal period is for women to receive compassionate, kind and dignifying care from their caregivers. I was so sad and appalled at the treatment of Shanay who was abducted from her garden and raped at the age of three:

'I had been in hospital four days. I used crutches even before labour, and then I had a third-degree tear. After birth, I was put in a suite around 2pm. I slept about seven hours straight after that. When I awoke, my husband had gone to the car. I was left in my room with my baby. Someone came round saying lunch was ready and I just needed to go down the aisle and get it. I asked her if she could bring me some. She said, "No, everyone else is getting their own food, so you should be able to. Besides, you've been in here a long time. You need to open the windows, get some fresh air and get some exercise." She left.

I hobbled to the door to catch her and said, "Please, I also don't want to leave my baby in here alone." She said, "Look at that queue, all these mums have left their babies in the room. Besides, we are around and nothing's going to happen."

I started choking up with tears in my eyes and she said, "Look, it's your birthday today, I hear. Consider it a test, if you can get your own breakfast, we will let you go home to celebrate your birthday." She walked away.

I clung on to the wall and began walking. I couldn't use the crutches because I wouldn't be able to carry my plate. Each step away from my room made me feel sick.

I was three years old when a man came into my garden, abducted me from my own home and raped me. This woman was telling me that people were watching. There wasn't even anyone at reception. And so many guys were walking in to come and see their partners, any one of them could have gone into my room and taken my baby. I am living proof of that.

As well as that, I, in all my pain and sickness, limping, crying, made it to the lunch table. Asked for something, tried to carry the plate and couldn't. I put it down. That same lady saw me. I left the plate and headed back to my room, feeling so terrible for leaving my baby.

The woman picked up my plate, rolled her eyes and gave a loud huff and brought the food to me. In my room, I wept and wept until my husband came. No words can describe what I felt

*and still feel. I don't think it's necessary for me to say what could
have been done better. The whole scenario is sickening.*

*Going forward, I think everyone who is going to be dealing
with mums needs to be educated, even receptionists, cleaners, etc.'*

I am convinced that had this caregiver come from a trauma-informed
approach, she would not have behaved in the way that she did. We
must assume that women have very good reasons for behaving the
way they do and for asking for the things they need.

Many survivors of abuse have such a traumatic time during labour
and birth that they consider not having any more children. Leila
explains:

*'I put off trying for another baby for a long time as the reality
was I wasn't sure if I could face that first year of having a baby
again. The guilt I felt at people telling me I should be enjoying it,
it's what I really wanted and the time goes so fast...when actually
for some of the time I was hating it. That felt a hard lesson to
have learnt.'*

When survivors have a positive experience there is so much that
can be healed in their body and mind. Georgia explains some of the
positive thoughts she had after the birth of her baby:

*'I actually felt a lot of confidence in my body post-partum too.
That was positive. Even though my body wasn't "perfect" I felt
really beautiful and in a place of acceptance (of my body). I felt
more confident 14 days postpartum than when I was 25 and
skinny.'*

Shanay feels that the birth of her baby moved her away from her past
and made her feel good about herself:

*'My birth was definitely healing as a new mum who had
struggled to conceive then had an anxious pregnancy. I believe*

the help of yoga, hypnobirthing and the shoulder to lean on with my doula were the perfect plan for a perfect birth. I am so very grateful my wishes were met and I was able to birth my baby into this world without thinking about my past.'

Paula feels extremely happy with her homebirth with the support of caring midwives and her husband:

'I learnt I could trust my body, that I was powerful, that I could do birth without being helped in any invasive way. Giving birth on all-fours felt so much more like I was in control – free to move without being tethered in any way increased my feelings of agency and independence and just helped the birth to flow more easily. The lack of interventions as a result of this bodily freedom is not just a nice bonus but was a turning point for me in believing in myself and finding in that moment true confidence as a powerful woman and mother.'

Summary

- Explore with a new mum any issues around breastfeeding and help her find solutions that will work for her.
- Reassure her that being a mother is not the romanticised picture we all have in our minds and that being a mum is challenging for everyone.
- Talk about 'good enough' parenting and that there is no such thing as a perfect mum.
- Remember that everyone is the way they are for a reason and you don't need to know why – everyone should be treated with kindness, dignity and respect.

Chapter 5

Healing Through Birth

When I asked the women who had filled out my questionnaire about sharing their positive birth stories, not everyone was able to contribute. Many survivors do not remember childbirth and motherhood as a healing experience at all. This is partly due to the lack of understanding of their specific needs but also due to a misunderstanding of their behaviour by staff. I believe, however, that this time in a woman's life is a great opportunity for her to start her recovery and that a positive experience of pregnancy, birth and the postnatal period can form an important part in the process of healing from sexual violence and re-claiming her body.

As you will see from the stories and as most survivors will explain, the past is not something that will ever go away and be forgotten but it is possible to put it to rest and move forward as a stronger and wiser person.

Paula's story

During my first pregnancy I was overjoyed that my body was doing something wholesome. After abuse at 13 from my own father, and a rather promiscuous teenhood (to drown out the memories of it) I was ready to feel healed and whole.

Unfortunately my planned homebirth was jeopardised by midwives who would not come out to assess me so after hours of painful contractions at home (back labour), I felt I had no other option but go to hospital – upon arrival I was assessed and told my cervix was 7 centimetres dilated. Wild horses couldn't drag me to get back in a car so I stayed at hospital and gave birth there.

There was no support to give birth actively whatsoever so I ended up in lithotomy on my back, all very disempowering and invasive.

I was mortifyingly embarrassed about being abused and I thought that by mentioning it, I was bringing the past to life and that was something I was desperate to put behind me. I didn't want to re-activate feelings of hopelessness at this precious and new point in my life.

After that birth it seemed everyone I knew had a more traumatic story than mine, ending in emergency caesareans with the baby 'nearly dying', so I swallowed my feelings and figured I got off 'lightly'.

Deep down, I blamed my birth on my own naivety but needed to feel good about it all, so it wouldn't spoil my first year with my son and leave me feeling traumatised. So I think minimising the horror of it became a strategy to help me be OK about it. And, I was so in love with being a mother and felt so natural and good so was on a high from how much I loved him and how easy my breastfeeding was.

After that, I was fortunate with excellent homebirth care and support from both GPs and midwives. The next two babies I had were easy and pleasurable by comparison to my hospital experience in terms of being in control of my own body, free to move, etc. Less VEs, and only performed by one midwife who I felt safe with. Again I never mentioned my abuse because I didn't want to spoil these special occasions, talking or thinking about the worst period of my life. These two births were truly healing.

Baby number four and in a new location, where I found myself having an unsupportive anti-homebirth GP, which was a shock and I felt a sense of grief that I was facing this birth in a spirit of 'going against medical advice' in spite of every indication, scan, measurement, etc. being perfect. This was a totally problem-free pregnancy. I had to be mentally strong and not rely on the NHS so much which made me feel resentful but determined. The midwife that turned up was faffing and a bit bossy. I turned very much inward and just focused on my body and gave birth on all fours with ease, in spite of her telling me not to push!

Baby number five, I ended up choosing to free-birth as my only other realistic option was hospital and I had had enough experience of what my own body could do by now to know I didn't want to hand it over to be handled roughly and more than necessary due to 'routine' hospital practices. I just wanted to do it quietly on my own, without drama, bright lights, stress, noise, lots of personalities and egos to have to assimilate alongside the power of contractions. I just wanted to be like a mammal and go on pure instincts.

I think by then I had just had enough of people behaving with authority and ownership over my own body. Now nearly 40 years old, I had simply had enough of that in my life.

Speaking about abuse for me only came after my birthing years. I think this was to avoid being re-traumatised. I wanted to keep it separate from the most beautiful thing in my life – my children. I very much wanted to keep the two things very much apart so as not to spoil my memories of their birth days.

Even now, I worry my children might find out about it while some of them are too young to be able to cope and process it, and part of me wants to preserve their innocence.

I think healthcare professionals need to assume that all mothers have been the subject of sexual violence or abuse and act with sensitivity. It's easier than putting the onus on mothers to tick a box, putting them on the spot – especially if they have other young children at the appointment – mothers shouldn't have to be re-traumatised just so healthcare professionals can switch into a different 'more sensitive' mode with that new knowledge about a mother. All women should receive the same, sensitive, gentle care, and respect.

Esme's story

With my second pregnancy I decided that I was not going to allow what happened the first time happen again and that I would have full control of my body, feelings and emotions. I was lucky enough to have the same midwife who supported me through my first birth and I also made my wishes clear to her.

I left it much later before going into hospital this time; I was watching 30-minute episodes of a box set and kept giving myself another episode before I went in.

I arrived at hospital and my cervix was a good few centimetres dilated and I was advised to walk around a bit more. They broke my waters which sent me into a panic and I started to freak out and wanted to leave as I thought this was going to go the same way as it did with my first baby. I was worried that they were going to make me do things to meet the clock again.

I managed to pull it together and completely calm down and with the help of some gas and air, I lay on the bed and got myself into a position I wanted to be in. Everyone was dosing off and the midwife was making notes at the end of the bed. I asked to just be left alone. They did a trace on my baby's heart tone and everything was fine. I was so exhausted in my first birth and wasted so much energy unnecessarily. This time, I had my earphones in and I didn't want to take them out or move to tell anyone when I felt bearing-down sensations so I decided to start pushing my baby down the birth canal.

I heard my husband get everyone's attention as he wanted to know what my stomach was doing. My mum was behind me and lifted my leg up and said to the midwife that she could see my baby's head crowning. I still just had my earphones in and my eyes closed. I didn't want the lights on. I didn't want to move.

I pretty much gave birth to my daughter all by myself and the midwife brought her up onto my tummy. It was so calm and it was that way as I had felt brave enough to ask for it to be like this.

I said to my mum minutes after the birth, 'Wow, I would do that again!' I completely listened to my body this time and not to any of the procedures. I let my body decide when I was doing things and I just let it wash over me. My midwife was so supportive of this as she saw what happened to me the first time I gave birth and I don't think she ever got over it.

I coped so much better postnatal this time too. With my first baby, I had a double episiotomy and so much bruising with forceps.

My baby was kept in hospital for a week in special care and I wasn't allowed to be with her. They gave her formula instead of waking me for a feed and I was devastated.

With my second baby, I had some stitches again but I wasn't sore like before. I dressed her myself, fed her and I showered myself and ate breakfast. Six hours later, we were discharged and I was tucked up in my own bed with my baby.

Gita's story

There was a light dusting of snow as I felt the first throbs and twinges of labour. The air was scented with the anticipation of blood, sweat and new life. However, it was not until a week later as my body was recovering from the worst cold I had experienced for years that I truly began to labour. This in itself, that even though my body was riddled with a cold, labour started, amazed me and reminded me of how incredible women's bodies and babies are.

I entered the winding labyrinth of my baby's birth with an open heart and relaxed intention. Re-claiming my body and being gentle with my many layers has been a life's work. I teach yoga pre- and postnatally and work as a doula, supporting women, so to me, birth is beautiful and natural when acknowledged and truly heard as a unique experience to the mother and baby dyad. During this pregnancy I had worked with Emily Housman, a midwife and dream birth practitioner, in preparation for the birth. Her use of imagery was very helpful and brought new awareness and healing for me.

I began deepening into my labour at home. It was to be a long and slow night as I moved between surges and vapour baths because I was still congested and unable to breathe freely due to my cold. By the morning I called my doula and midwife for support. I was blessed that we all shared a deep knowing and trust in each other. I'd seen Paula for all of my antenatal appointments during this pregnancy and had known Thea, my doula, for some time. Without having planned this in advance, I was experiencing continuity of care and the deep trust this had established supported me to find trust in my body. I felt truly held.

My husband was my rock. He was holding me when I needed him the most and caring for our first born when he needed to be loved too. Those present witnessed me and trusted me in my own knowing. I requested a vaginal examination and was surprised to find that my cervix was 7 centimetres dilated, according to the medical model.

The intensity of my labour began to shift in unpredictable ways. Another couple of hours later and I began feeling beyond the edge. My body was aching with the symptoms of my cold and my older son was expressing distress. I was vomiting every bit of substance I'd tried eating and drinking. I wanted to transfer to hospital, get some hydration and some rest, as well as some relief from my back to back labour and then be able to welcome my baby earth side.

I felt very clear in my needs and intentions. Paula expressed how she wasn't concerned for the wellbeing of me or my baby, and Thea continued to offer support to help turn my baby into a more optimal position. I knew in my body that I wasn't feeling OK; this was confirmed by a raised temperature so I requested an examination which confirmed I'd stalled at 7 centimetres dilated.

Arriving at Torbay hospital was like arriving at a temple. The care and compassion of the midwives is beyond words to me. I waved a sweet cheerio to my midwife Paula and journeyed onwards with Thea. The same sensitivity and respect based on my background and birth preferences continued at the hospital.

After the support of a lot of hydration and a gentle epidural to soften the edge of my labour it was becoming apparent that my baby was ready to be born. I could feel him kicking off my ribs as my pelvis opened. Thea had suggested a fascia release earlier and within moments my son rotated and moved into the birth canal.

I felt strong, empowered and in control. However, there was a re-surfacing of my story that I didn't anticipate meeting in a non-emergency situation. The midwife informed me there was only a male doctor on the ward and that it was desirable for him to examine me to confirm my baby's positioning and my progress.

I felt myself freeze, tears streamed that I couldn't hold back. I felt invaded and a resurgence of raw emotion from my life's story. It wasn't OK and I heard myself offering to conform to allowing a man I didn't know to enter my body. I was drawing on all of my own inner resource to allow this to be OK. However, it simply wasn't. Thankfully I didn't need to voice this as the midwife caring for me sought out a female consultant who was finishing her shift on the day unit below.

This consultant chose to see me rather than go home on time. And for her presence I will always be grateful. Her examination confirmed what I was feeling in my body. My baby was ready to journey earth side. And so within three hours of arriving in hospital I was hydrated, feeling strong and pushing my son earth side. It was exhilarating, hard work and beautiful birthing my baby.

Georgia's story

One morning I woke up to find myself feeling wet. I was a bit confused, as pregnancy often had me. Was it discharge? Had I accidentally wet myself? I didn't think much of it, so I continued lying in bed just relaxing a bit, before I felt another little trickle. This time I thought: uh-oh, could it be my waters? But I was only 36 weeks pregnant, I thought. I went to the bathroom to find my underwear pretty soaked, but still I wasn't sure. Deep down I think I knew, but I couldn't trust my intuition in that moment. Throughout pregnancy I had had so many unfamiliar fluids. I told my husband, who was getting ready to go to work. I called my mum to talk it through with her. It seemed more likely it could've been my waters. I emailed my midwife to let her know, feeling super relaxed. She called me immediately laughing at the fact I had emailed her about my waters breaking so calmly. We decided to wait and see how the day went and if any contractions started.

I called a friend and asked if she wanted to go for brunch. It was a snowy December day in Manhattan and I set out to meet her. We sat and ate some food and I waited for any sign of labour. I called on my small team of support for help, my mum, my best friend, my doula and my homeopath. I was told to go and buy some broth and a cup with a straw and stay hydrated while I relaxed on all fours. It felt very serene.

By the end the day, my husband returned home from work and we called our midwife to let her know there was no sign of labour. She informed me that if nothing started during the night, we should meet her with our bags at the hospital the following morning to induce labour. I agreed and went to bed feeling excited, nervous and really not sure what to expect. In hindsight I really had no idea what it meant to be induced. All I knew was that my mum had to be induced while birthing me.

I slept as well as I could, which wasn't very well at all because I kept waking up to check if I could maybe be in labour, and anticipating how it would all go. We headed to meet the midwife in the morning and I remember feeling such a sense of calm. In the waiting room there was a woman in apparent labour and they were playing an episode of *Friends* where Phoebe was giving birth. I thought to myself: how powerful women are.

The nurse gave me an IV for the Pitocin, after my midwife had come in to check that my waters had really broken. Indeed they had, and she explained it was a high water breakage where the waters leak; however, in my case, labour hadn't started so they had to induce me as a precaution. They took us to our room and gave me an enema as I would soon be attached to the IV drip and therefore not able to move very far, and only able to reach a bedpan.

My mum came to meet us at the hospital which I wanted, and soon afterwards my doula arrived. We all sat in the room and chatted and laughed. I remember feeling glad of the conversation but also in this amazing world of my own. It felt as though there was a bubble around me. My doula raised the hospital bed so I could be sitting very high up, and lifted my back up so it was like a throne. The nurses kept coming in to check the monitors, which were showing my contractions were starting, but still I felt nothing. Hours passed. My doula got me to nap, and to meditate following a lovely birthing meditation. I drank apple juice and water with ice. Still, I felt calm. In the evening I started to feel some period-like cramps. My doula had me lie in different positions with the peanut ball. My husband napped, and went to get a burrito. One nurse kept coming in to check the monitors and she was really rubbing me the wrong way. Her energy wasn't making me feel relaxed but more nervous and not heard. My doula recognised this, and when it came time to push, I noticed that nurse was not the one to come in to assist.

After 15 hours of being induced, barely feeling any contractions but more period-like cramps, my midwife decided to break the rest of my bag of waters. As soon as they burst, my whole body and mind shifted. I felt the desperate need to throw up and then afterwards to pee. My midwife and doula seemed excited and pleased by this and were so encouraging. My energy became much less internal and it was as though it was all pouring out of me. As I sat down to pee on the bedpan, I could feel the rush of the first contraction. It was as though the contraction would speed up and then hit a peak, where I would breathe through and make these animalistic noises which would help me get through, and then there would be a break. These noises came out of my mouth involuntarily, and I was embarrassed at how they sounded. I felt the need to bear down, leaning and swaying on the birth ball while my doula and husband put cold compresses on my neck, back and head. My midwife crouched behind me while she watched my progress, and my mum sat on a chair in the corner. Everyone in the room had a presence that was perfectly subtle. Nobody was overwhelming, only quietly supportive. After several of these contractions, during a break, I asked the room if they thought maybe I should get an epidural. I didn't demand one; I just wanted to hear their opinion. I wanted to hear them say I was going to be OK and I could get through it. My mum told me the best thing I wanted to hear at that moment; she said, 'It won't get any worse than this.' That I could manage, I thought, if I have got through those ones, I can get through these.

My legs started to feel a bit weak, and I told my midwife that my daughter was coming and I wanted to lie down because I felt a bit too tired to be standing. It felt like ten minutes of contractions had passed but I know now that it was about an hour. When I was on the bed the midwife asked me to see if being on all fours felt good, but I didn't like that, so I lay on my back. Once I was in this position, I felt the strong urge of my body pushing my daughter out. It was amazing to experience my body doing everything for me. All I needed to do was really just let go and embrace what my body knew so well to do. That was a hard thing for me to do, to let go. The pushes felt overwhelming but I remember the smiles of my midwife and the nurse, holding up my legs and encouraging me to keep going and saying that I was doing great. It burned around my vagina as my daughter's head came out, and my midwife asked if I wanted to reach down to look at her head but I really didn't want to, I felt scared. After a few more pushes, her body came gushing out and she was on my chest in my arms. She was calm and beautiful and she was finally here. Those moments still sometimes feel like a dream to me. There is a part of me that can't believe that she and I went on that journey together.

Birthing the placenta felt so satisfying. With a little push, it came out, and the journey felt complete. My baby was in my arms, and I felt like a superhero having just given birth. I asked my mum to order me a milkshake and fries, and my husband, my baby and I all held each other.

Ellen's story

When I found myself pregnant with my sixth child I knew I couldn't have a repeat of the previous five pregnancies where I felt let down by the system. I didn't want to have to explain my complex history at each appointment or feel coerced into interventions I didn't want. I didn't want to leave each appointment feeling as if my consent wasn't sought, as a PTSD sufferer due to past abuse; it really is a horrible feeling.

My fourth pregnancy was my first with my now husband. He is extremely loving and supportive, the complete opposite of my previous partner. I didn't think that my past experiences would impact on me as I was now in a safe loving environment but it hit me hard and my anxiety peaked, my mental health struggled at times, especially when I found out I was expecting a son. I went into panic mode on how I could possibly raise a boy to turn into a caring man and not an abusive one. It took a good few sessions with my psychologist to change my thought process. His birth was an induction due to hospital error which had its own issues and he ended up in the neonatal intensive care unit (NICU). I felt helpless and I felt guilty that he was born naturally, like I had tainted him by letting him pass through the area where I was abused. I sat sobbing with my psychologist over it but I was struck with this overwhelming love and need to protect my son. He came to me for a reason and it was to heal me.

I quickly found myself pregnant again and discovered that it was another boy. I was so happy about it but found myself up against opposition at the hospital. I was repeatedly told 'no' to all my requests around the birth and it has a huge impact on my PTSD. I felt my rights were being removed, that this baby was no longer mine. I enlisted the help of Birthrights (an organisation to protect human rights in maternity) and with them on my side, I fought for a homebirth from 36 weeks of pregnancy. My son didn't wait for the midwives to arrive and he was born with just his dad in the room. The midwives were so respectful of my wants and wishes and my birth space. It was an amazing experience and one I felt was healing. I felt a newfound love for my body.

Along came baby number six and this time I didn't want a fight. I had my booking-in appointment at eight weeks where I declined any further antenatal appointments. I did agree to telephone calls with one community midwife at the same time as regular check-ups. I also let the Head of Midwifery know I would be seeking homebirth support from 36 weeks as I wanted the homebirth kit dropped off just in case. My intention was also to call them after the birth but I wanted to birth alone. I read a lot of birth books, I fully submerged myself in the 'free-birthing' world and I believed my body and mind could do it. I wanted to give birth to my baby without any medical personnel present.

I hit a couple of bumps in the road where I found myself in the triage area of the hospital. While there, I felt bullied and given every scare story by doctors to get me to agree to their way. I could have crumbled but I didn't. Even the day I had Ingrid I found myself in triage being told my baby and myself could die unless I did exactly as they said. The language used and the threats really pushed me into a PTSD anxiety attack. My heart was racing, I was holding back tears, I wanted to run away and hide, I felt so scared by the man in front of me telling me I was stupid for not agreeing with him. I don't know how, maybe it was the inbuilt protective mother, but I found the courage to ask for a second opinion. His senior arrived and she talked over everything with me, told me to go home and rest as labour was near. Getting home and into my protected space with my loved ones was what I needed.

I had the most amazing free-birth with only my husband in the room. It all happened so quickly. I sat forward on the sofa at 10.06pm while laughing at the TV and felt a gush of fluids. I went to the toilet and said I would head to bed to sleep for a bit of rest. I got upstairs and climbed into bed but I instantly made my way back downstairs and calmly told my husband not to bother with the pool as our daughter was coming quickly. I perched myself on the edge of the sofa and moaned through the following few surges. I needed the quiet this time. I then felt the urge to lie on the sofa, the exact same as I had with her brother just ten months earlier. Within three quick surges, my baby's head began to crown. I reached down to touch her head and then moved my hands out the way. Her head was birthed followed by her body with the next surge and her dad placed his hands to welcome her to the world and put her onto me. She was perfect.

My husband and I connected on a whole new level, and he kept me grounded and kept the space protected as I breathed our baby out. It was the most mesmerising, uplifting, spiritual experience I could have wished for. I felt like a warrior woman and yet I felt calm. She entered the world to quiet stillness. We were at peace. The midwives arrived and gave us time but we needed a transfer into hospital as she had slightly laboured breathing. From there on I was once again at the mercy of the medical team that surrounded me, I found the NICU journey a struggle because of this imbalance of power, my mood did decline, PTSD peaked but I had my husband and children around me to keep me strong.

Here I am expecting another baby; I have opted out of maternity care and plan on free-birthing again. Having PTSD makes this journey so much harder; the maternity world is tough to navigate and an innocent comment can leave you feeling scared and open up wounds. I don't want to risk that happening too often so I am stepping back and taking control. I believe that, however you choose to birth, it's important to surround yourself with people who understand your needs and can protect your birth space. It makes the difference between having a bad experience and a positive empowering one.

Conclusion

I have to say that writing this book has been a humbling experience and also one of the hardest things I've ever done. I felt an immense pressure to make this important book the best it could be. I now kind of understand why this book has not been written before. It's upsetting to hear how women every day have disappointing and upsetting experiences that could have been prevented if someone that was looking after them had been kind.

I've studied with some very prominent people in the field looking at how to support survivors better and I've read numerous books, research papers and articles. During my time working as a birth doula, I've supported many survivors through labour and birth, and, generally speaking, applied most of what I learnt about supporting survivors to everyone that I've ever supported. The subject of abuse is still a social taboo; even though we talk about it more and see it discussed in social media, there is still a resistance to getting maternity workers on training courses and workshops. It's often viewed as a dark and deep subject which could upset everyone. It can, of course, also trigger memories of abuse for anyone attending and as we know sexual abuse and violence are widespread, that is very likely to be the case. I wonder sometimes if we don't want to learn more about this because we worry about how it's going to affect us. It can be scary to dig deep into our own pasts and also to learn of the many things that we as maternity workers may have done to women in our care that would have caused harm. What I do know is that we must start taking this issue seriously and we must start putting education in place for all maternity workers so that we can support women better.

I've learnt so much from the women who helped me write this book by filling out my questionnaire and sharing their harrowing accounts of the abuse they survived and the impact it had on the birth of their babies, as well as beyond that. I'm forever grateful for their help and support and willingness to make this book a reality in the hope that women in the future who enter maternity services will have more compassionate care and come through the other end stronger and empowered from what they have achieved. It is only by listening to the women themselves that we can learn how to best support them.

All women deserve dignity, respect and kindness during the child-bearing years but survivors of sexual abuse need this in abundance. They have been badly let down already, often by someone that they should have been able to trust and rely on, someone that they might have loved as well. The trauma and damage this has caused to their trust and belief in others is unimaginable. The overarching feelings they have grown up with, shame, disgust, anger and fear, cannot and must not be overlooked or ignored by anyone, especially someone in maternity care who is there to celebrate one of the best days of this woman's life, the birth of her baby. All women must be given evidence-based information in an unbiased and non-confrontational way so that they can make choices for themselves and their babies. We must change the paternalistic maternity system that often over-rides what women are feeling and wanting for themselves. I realise that many healthcare professionals might worry about litigation and accusations if their recommendations are not followed and the baby or mother is harmed in some way as a result. However, in my view, one thing follows on from the other. If women are listened to and kindly treated, fewer of them will be unhappy about their experience and this would lead to less litigation. I really do believe that steamrolling women into doing what you think is best as a healthcare professional will not prevent litigation – it is more likely to cause it. We must look at the real risks involved with childbirth, which overall are no greater than other things we do in life, if a woman is well and healthy in her pregnancy.

There is plenty of research that shows survivors of abuse will be suffering from PTSD as well as other trauma symptoms. We also know that when our nervous system is regularly stimulated in intense and unpredictable ways, it become over-sensitive. This means that tiny stimulations which would not cause much of a reaction in a healthy system can elicit extreme activation of the nervous system. The brain could be telling survivors that they are under attack even though there is no apparent threat or danger. Their baseline of alarm is different from someone who is not a survivor which means they will be thinking, behaving and acting differently. It is not for anyone else to judge situations as being traumatising or not as this can only be for the person experiencing the event to know. It's therefore important to always check in with women who are coming through maternity services whether procedures and guidelines are going to be triggering for them or cause trauma.

Growing up in an environment that is unsafe also impacts on the child's development of the capacity to trust, to be intimate, to feel autonomy and also on their sexuality. Mullen and Fleming (1998) referred to these mental health problems, connected to the history of abuse, as second-order effects. This is what makes a difference between survivors of sexual violence as adults and survivors of childhood sexual abuse. A study that looked at adult women who were survivors of childhood sexual abuse discovered that the women who had been abused over a more extended time and multiple times displayed more elevated levels of psychological problems when compared with those that had been abused only once in their life (Banyard, Williams and Siegel 2001).

Another finding worth noting is that women who are survivors of CSA are more prone to sexual and physical violence later in their lives. One study in Australia showed that the risk was one and a half times higher, from 29 per cent to 43 per cent, when compared to women who were not survivors of sexual abuse (Mouzos and Makkai 2004).

There are a number of recognisable behaviours in survivors of sexual abuse and sexual violence although just because someone is displaying some of these, it doesn't automatically mean that they are survivors. Any kind of trauma in a woman's past is going to have an impact on the way she is behaving and shape the person she becomes. However, all women should be treated with compassion, respect and kindness as the likelihood of previous sexual violence or childhood abuse is statistically pretty high (as discussed above).

Healthcare professionals are always asking questions and taking samples to look out for medical conditions or obstetric emergencies, when, in fact, they are much more likely to be supporting a survivor. The most common pregnancy complication is pre-eclampsia, which occurs in around 6 per cent of pregnancies and preterm birth, affecting 7–8 per cent of pregnant women and their babies (Tommys 2019a, 2019b). In comparison, some UK studies indicate that around 20 per cent of women are survivors of sexual abuse and this, in my opinion, is very likely just the top of the iceberg (as discussed in Chapter 1).

Still, there are no universal procedures to find out about this or clinical guidelines on how to deal with it. I guess it opens up a kind of Pandora's Box as there needs to be more support for healthcare professionals for them to be able to sensitively deal with this as well as get support for themselves. In an already overstretched NHS, where everyone is working at top capacity, just about able to cope with the current situation, I fear this could simply tip it all over the edge.

However, in my view, what we can no longer allow is for women to enter the maternity system relatively healthy and come out the other end broken or even completely shattered by their experience. There should be a lot fewer women having to deal with PTSD and other mental health problems when they have just become mothers. We talk about support for mental health, both perinatal and postnatal, but what if there was a way of minimising the risks of postnatal illness from the beginning? What if we could provide better and more dignified care to the women who we meet and by doing so, prevent the mental health issues in the first place? If women were better supported during childbirth, if women were having positive experiences, feeling part of the decision-making, and feeling seen and heard, I truly believe we would prevent a huge number of new mums experiencing mental health problems.

In my view, there is only one way of achieving this and it's not a new idea or even my idea but women must be put at the centre of the care. If each and every one of us put all our perceived and perhaps even real differences away, removed the ego of each care provider and put all our energy and focus into making each maternity experience the best it can be for each woman we meet, I believe we could achieve something wonderful.

I feel that a lot of the fundamental problems are down to the demands of the institutions which force caregivers to focus more on guidelines and protocols, rather than each woman's individual needs. The woman becomes a disembodiment, an object, deprived of feelings and authority, which leads to invasive medical procedures, such as vaginal examination and suturing of vaginal tears, sometimes being carried out without compassion or with disregard of how these things will impact on the woman's mental health. Instead of listening to what women are saying, they become vessels to be safely emptied of their precious goods with the thought that any psychological damage or trauma can be fixed later. To look after a woman's mental health might be seen as not part of the job description for maternity workers; that belongs in the mental health department, which women can be referred to later. Perhaps there is a false belief that everything will be forgiven and forgotten if both the mother and the baby are alive. This is, of course, important but we might need to start putting a woman's psychological health and wellbeing in the same place in terms of priorities. We might need to stop viewing clinical guidelines and procedures as top of the list and make it just as important to offer a human connection and value emotional interaction with the birthing woman, especially during births that take place on labour wards in hospitals as the focus is often quite different on midwifery-led units and amongst homebirth teams in the community.

There is still a lot of work to be done in terms of educating maternity care workers in the human rights around childbirth. A woman's autonomy and right to make choices for herself and her baby need to be reiterated again and again. Women do not take these decisions lightly and will often be well read and educated on the topic. In an article written by Rebecca Schiller, she quotes a senior obstetrician (who wished to remain anonymous) saying 'There isn't enough understanding of the basic medical ethical principle of the right to autonomy.' The same obstetrician followed on by saying that there is 'clear evidence that women's right to make their own informed choices is not clearly understood' (Schiller 2016).

I believe the very reason women are making some choices is because they have come to the conclusion that it is the right and safest choice in their minds. If all choices are based on the available research and the risks have been weighed up, the choices of a woman should be honoured and respected. There are not choices that are 100 per cent safe! It must always be up to the woman to decide what perceived risks she is willing to take.

Medical interventions and routine procedures all carry some risk but when we talk about childbirth, we know from the extensive Birth Place Study (Birthplace in England Collaborative Group 2011) that statistically, if a woman is having a healthy pregnancy, it is 99.57 per cent likely that she and her baby will be absolutely fine. Maternal death is very rare in the UK but does vary, depending on ethnic background. The report, *Saving Lives, Improving Mothers' Care*, by MBRRACE-UK published in 2018 shows that the risks are 8 in 100,000 if you are a white woman, 15 in 100,000 if you are an Asian woman and 40 in 100,000 if you are a black woman. There is an urgent and great need to gain more understanding and research into why there are such differences. The report highlighted that most women who died had multiple health problems as well as other vulnerabilities, such as addiction, abuse or domestic violence.

It often feels like maternity services are driven by fear and everyone involved is fearful of what is a physiological and natural event. Somehow we have managed to survive and reproduce for 3 million years, if we consider Lucy as our first ancestor. (Lucy was discovered in 1974 in Africa; she is an early australopithecine and one of the most important fossils ever discovered.) I'm pretty sure there have always been doulas and midwives involved in supporting at births and there is a mountain of research suggesting that this is still the safest and best way for healthy pregnant women to be supported (Sandall *et al.* 2016; McRae *et al.* 2018; Sehhatie *et al.* 2014).

Obstetrics are helping a lot of women with complex needs but that is where it should stay. Obstetric care should not be routine for women who do not need the support of someone who often, from my understanding, has not had much experience with supporting at physiological births and who is usually called upon only when there is a problem.

We are at risk of losing the most important skills that midwives bring, the emotional and practical support, that is now often complemented by doulas who offer this as their only focus. If you understand birth physiology, then you know that protecting the space for a woman to shut down her neo-cortex and tune into the primitive part of her brain is very important for a straightforward birth. If this is lost in the fear-driven focus on clinical guidelines and paperwork, we really are standing at a juncture that would drive maternity care down a completely medicalised route, robbing women of the opportunity to experience the miracle and empowerment of giving birth naturally. It would deprive women who are survivors of childhood sexual abuse as well as sexual violence the opportunity to reclaim their body and find admiration for it again.

My call to action is for everyone involved in maternity care and supporting women during what can be a very vulnerable time, especially for survivors of sexual abuse and violence, to evaluate our different roles and to go back to basics. What really makes a difference for women is the presence of someone who is listening to them, caring for them and including them in all the discussions. Every woman needs to feel loved and cared for during pregnancy, childbirth and in the postnatal period. Yes, we need professionalism and boundaries but that doesn't mean we have to stop being human beings: human beings connecting with other human beings, emotionally and empathetically.

All women who choose to engage with maternity care must come out the other end with their dignity and autonomy still intact. We all need to do more to ensure woman-centred care is happening in all the hospitals across the land.

No woman should come away from pregnancy and childbirth without awe and pride in her achievements and completely in love with her baby.

It all starts with you – I invite you to become part of the solution!

References

Alvarez-Segura, M., Garcia-Esteve, L., Torres, A., Plaza, A., Imaz, M.L., Hermida-Barros, L., San, L. and Burtchen, N. (2014) 'Are women with a history of abuse more vulnerable to perinatal depressive symptoms? A systematic review.' *Archives of Women's Mental Health 17*, 5, 343–57.

Banyard, V.L., Williams, L.M. and Siegel, JA. (2001) 'The long-term mental health consequences of child sexual abuse: an exploratory study of the impact of multiple traumas in a sample of women.' *Journal of Traumatic Stress 14*, 4, 697–715.

Benedict, M.I., Paine, L. and Paine, L. (1994) *Long-term Effects of Sexual Abuse in Childhood on Psychosocial Functioning in Pregnancy and Pregnancy Outcome.* Washington, DC: Department of Health and Human Services National Center on Child Abuse and Neglect.

Benedict, M.I., Paine, L.L., Paine, L.A., Brandt, D. and Stallings, R. (1999) 'The association of childhood sexual abuse with depressive symptoms during pregnancy, and selected pregnancy outcomes.' *Child Abuse & Neglect 23*, 7, 659–70.

Berman, H., Mason, R., Hall, J. Rodger, S., Classen, C.C., Evans, M.K., Ross, L.E., Alvernaz Mulcahy, G., Carranza, L. and Al-Zoubi, F. (2014) 'Laboring to mother in the context of past trauma: the transition to motherhood.' *Qualitative Health Research 24*, 9, 1253–64.

Bohren, M.A., Hofmeyr, G., Sakala, C., Fukuzawa, R.K. and Cuthbert, A. (2017) 'Continuous support for women during childbirth.' *Cochrane Database of Systematic Reviews 7*. Art. No.: CD003766.

Brener, N.D., McMahon, P.M., Warren, C.W. and Douglas, K.A. (1999) 'Forced sexual intercourse and associated health-risk behaviors among female college students in the United States.' *Journal of Consulting and Clinical Psychology 67*, 2, 252–9.

Briere, J. N. and Elliot, D. (1994) 'Immediate and long-term impacts of child sexual abuse.' *Future Child 4*, 2, 54–69.

Calero, H.H. (2005) *The Power of Nonverbal Communication: How You Act Is More Important Than What You Say (Taking Control).* Aberdeen: Silver Lake Publishing.

Centre for Action on Rape and Abuse (2016) 'What is sexual violence?' Accessed on 2/8/18 at https://caraessex.org.uk/whatissexualviolence.php.

Coles, J., Anderson, A. and Loxton, D. (2016) 'Breastfeeding duration after childhood sexual abuse: an Australian cohort study.' *Journal of Human Lactation 32*, 3, 28–35.

Courtois, C.A. (1996) *Healing the Incest Wound: Adult Survivors in Therapy.* New York: W.W. Norton & Company.

Devane, D., Lalor, J.G., Daly, S., McGuire, W., Cuthbert, A. and Smith, V. (2017) 'Cardiotocography versus intermittent auscultation of fetal heart on admission to labour ward for assessment of fetal wellbeing.' *The Cochrane Database of Systematic Reviews 26.*

Douglas, A.R. (2000) 'Reported anxieties concerning intimate parenting in women sexually abused as children.' *Child Abuse & Neglect 24*, 425–34.

Elfgen, C., Hagenbuch, N., Görres, G., Block, E. and Leeners, B. (2017) 'Breastfeeding in women having experienced childhood sexual abuse.' *Journal of Human Lactation 33*, 1, 119–27.

Egeland, B., Jacobvitz, D. and Sroufe, L.A. (1988) 'Breaking the cycle of abuse.' *Child Development 59*, 4, 1080–8.

Erickson, M. (1976) 'The relationship between psychological variables and specific complications of pregnancy, labor, and delivery.' *Journal of Psychosomatic Research 20*, 3, 207–10.

Garratt, L. (2010) *Survivors of Childhood Sexual Abuse and Midwifery Practice.* Abingdon: Radcliffe Publishing Ltd.

Glasser, M., Kolvin, I., Campbell, D., Glasser, A., Leitch, I. and Farrelly, S. (2001) 'Cycle of child sexual abuse: links between being a victim and becoming a perpetrator.' *British Journal of Psychiatry 179*, 6, 482–94.

Grimstad, H. and Schei, B. (1999) 'Pregnancy and delivery for women with a history of child sexual abuse.' *Child Abuse & Neglect 23*, 1, 81–90.

Halldórsdóttir, S. and Karlsdóttir, S.I. (1996) 'Empowerment or discouragement: women's experience of caring and uncaring encounters during childbirth.' *Health Care for Women International 17*, 4, 361–79.

Häuser, W., Kosseva, M., Üceyler, N., Klose, P. and Sommer, C. (2011) 'Emotional, physical, and sexual abuse in fibromyalgia syndrome: a systematic review with meta-analysis.' *Arthritis Care & Research 63*, 6, 808–20.

Heidt, J.M., Marxa, B.P. and Forsyth, J.P. (2005) 'Tonic immobility and childhood sexual abuse: a preliminary report evaluating the sequela of rape-induced paralysis.' *Behaviour Research and Therapy 43*, 9, 1157–71.

Heimstad, R., Dahloe, R., Laache, I., Skogvoll, E. and Schei B. (2006) 'Fear of childbirth and history of abuse: implications for pregnancy and delivery.' *Acta Obstetricia et Gynecologica 85*, 435–40.

Henriksen, L., Schei, B., Vangen, S. and Lukasse, M. (2014) 'Sexual violence and mode of delivery: a population-based cohort study.' *BJOG 121*, 10, 1237–44.

Herman, J. (1997) *Trauma and Recovery: The Aftermath of Violence – From Domestic Abuse to Political Terror.* New York: Basic Books.

Huhn, K.A. and Brost, B.C. (2004) 'Accuracy of simulated cervical dilation and effacement measurements among practitioners.' *American Journal of Obstetrics and Gynacology 191*, 5, 1797–9.

Iribarren, J., Prolo, P., Neagos, N. and Chiappelli, F. (2005) 'Post-Traumatic Stress Disorder: evidence-based research for the third millennium.' *Evidence-Based Complementary and Alternative Medicine 2*, 4, 503–12.

Kaufman, J. and Zigler, E. (1987) 'Do abused children become abusive parents?' *American Journal of Orthopsychiatry 57*, 2, 186–92.

Lang, A.J., Rodgers, C.S., Laffaye, C., Satz, L.E., Dresselhaus, T.R. and Stein, M.B. (2010) 'Sexual trauma, posttraumatic stress disorder, and health behaviour.' *Behavioral Medicine 28*, 4, 150–58.

Leeners, B., Richter-Appelt, H., Imthurn, B. and Rath, W. (2006) 'Influence of childhood sexual abuse on pregnancy, delivery, and the early postpartum period in adult women.' *Journal of Psychosomatic Research 61*, 2, 139–51.

Leeners, B., Stiller, R., Block, E., Görres, G., Imthurn, B. and Rath, W. (2007) 'Effect of childhood sexual abuse on gynecologic care as an adult.' *Psychosomatics 48*, 5, 385–93.

Leeners, B., Stiller, R., Block, E., Görres, G. and Rath W. (2010) 'Pregnancy complications in women with childhood sexual abuse experiences.' *Journal of Psychosomatic Research 69*, 503–10.

Lukasse, M., Henriksen, L., Vangen, S. and Schei, B. (2012) 'Sexual violence and pregnancy-related physical symptoms.' *BMC Pregnancy and Childbirth 12*, 83.

Lukasse, M., Vangen, S., Øian, P., Kumle, M., Ryding, E.L. and Schei, B. (2009) 'Childhood abuse and fear of childbirth: a population-based study.' *Birth 37*, 4, 267–74.

McRae, D.N., Janssen, P.A., Vedam, S., Mayhew, M., Mpofu, D., Teucher, U. and Muhajarine, N. (2018) 'Reduced prevalence of small-for-gestational-age and preterm birth for women of low socioeconomic position: a population-based cohort study comparing antenatal midwifery and physician models of care.' *BMJ Open 8*, 10.

MBRRACE-UK (2018) *Saving Lives, Improving Mothers' Care*. November. MBRRACE-UK.

Mehrabian, A. (1972) *Nonverbal Communication*. New York: Transaction Publishers.

Möller, A., Söndergaard, H.P. and Helström, L. (2017) 'Tonic immobility during sexual assault – a common reaction predicting post-traumatic stress disorder and severe depression.' *Acta Obstetricia et Gynecologica Scandinavica 96*, 8, 932–38.

Montgomery, E. (2013) 'Feeling safe: a metasynthesis of the maternity care needs of women who were sexually abused in childhood.' *Birth: Issues in Perinatal Care 40*, 2, 88–95.

Mouzos, J. and Makkai, T. (2004) 'Women's experience of male violence: findings from the Australian Component of the International Violence against Women Survey.' Australian Institute of Criminology. Accessed on 28/11/18 at www.ncjrs. gov/App/Publications/abstract.aspx?ID=208354.

Mullen, P. and Fleming, J. (1998) 'Long-term effects of child sexual abuse.' *Issues in Child Abuse Prevention 9*, Australian Institute of Family Studies. Accessed on 31/11/18 at https://aifs.gov.au/cfca/publications/long-term-effects-child-sexual-abuse-1998.

Nelson, S. and Phillips, S. (2001) *Beyond Trauma: Mental Health Care Needs of Women Who Survived Childhood Sexual Abuse*. Health in Mind.

Nerum, H., Halvorsen, L., Sørlie, T. and Øian, P. (2006) 'Maternal request for cesarean section due to fear of birth: can it be changed through crisis-oriented counseling?' *Birth 33*, 3, 221–8.

Nerum, H., Halvorsen, L., Straume, B., Sørlie, T. and Øian, P. (2013) 'Different labour outcomes in primiparous women that have been subjected to childhood sexual abuse or rape in adulthood: a case-control study in a clinical cohort.' *BJOG: An International Journal of Obstetrics and Gynaecology 120*, 4, 487–95.

NHS England (2019) *Perinatal.* Accessed on 28/6/19 at www.england.nhs.uk/mental-health/perinatal.

Noll, J.G., Horowitz, L.A., Bonanno, G.A., Trickett, P.K. and Putnam, F.W. (2003) 'Revictimization and self-harm in females who experienced childhood sexual abuse: results from a prospective study.' *Journal of Interpersonal Violence 18*, 12, 1452–71.

O'Connell, M.A., Leahy-Warren, P., Khashan ,A.S., Kenny, L.C. and O'Neill, S.M. (2017) 'Worldwide prevalence of tocophobia in pregnant women: systematic review and meta-analysis.' *Acta Obstetricia et Gynecologica Scandinavica 96*, 8, 907–20.

Office for National Statistics (2017) Sexual offences in England and Wales: year ending March 2017. Accessed on 2/8/18 at www.ons.gov.uk/peoplepopulation andcommunity/crimeandjustice/articles/sexualoffencesinenglandandwales/ yearendingmarch2017.

Prentice, J.C., Lu, M.C., Lange, L. and Halfton, N. (2002) 'The association between reported childhood sexual abuse and breastfeeding initiation.' *Journal of Human Lactation 18*, 3, 219–26.

Radford, L., Corral, S., Bradley, C., Fisher, H., Bassett, C., Howat, N. and Collishaw, S. (2011) *Child Abuse and Neglect in the UK Today.* London: NSPCC.

Raphael, D. (1976) *The Tender Gift: Breast Feeding.* New York: Schocken Books.

RCM (2017) 'Act now to avert growing crisis in our maternity services.' 6 February. Accessed on 23/6/19 at www.rcm.org.uk/media-releases/2017/february/act-now-to-avert-growing-crisis-in-our-maternity-services-says-rcm-as-it-launches-its-latest-report.

Repi, T. (2008) *Nemi Kriki Spolne Zlorabe in Novo Upanje (The Silent Cry of Sexual Abuse and a New Hope).* Založba Mohorjeva Družba: Celje.

Riggs, D.S., Murdock, T. and Walsh, W. (1992) 'A prospective examination of post-traumatic stress disorder in rape victims.' *Journal of Traumatic Stress 5*, 3, 455–75.

Rodgers, C.S., Lang, A.J., Twamley, E.W. and Stein, M.B. (2003) 'Sexual trauma and pregnancy: a conceptual framework.' *Journal of Women's Health 12*, 10, 961–70.

Royal College of Obstetrics and Gynaecologists (2015) 'Clinical Governance Advice No. 6.' RCOG. Accessed on 29/2/19 at www.rcog.org.uk/globalassets/documents/ guidelines/clinical-governance-advice/cga6.pdf.

Ruscio, A.M. (2001) 'Predicting the child-rearing practices of mothers sexually abused in childhood.' *Child Abuse & Neglect*, 25, 369–87.

Sachs, A. (2018) 'A new way to think about the transition to motherhood.' TED talk. Accessed on 29/2/19 at www.ted.com/talks/alexandra_sacks_a_new_way_to_ think_about_the_transition_to_motherhood.

Saisto, T., Kaaja, R., Ylikorkala, O. and Halmesmaki, E. (2001) 'Reduced pain tolerance during and after pregnancy in women suffering from fear of labor.' *Pain 93*, 2, 123–7.

Sandall, J., Soltani, H., Gates, S., Shennan, A. and Devane, D. (2016) 'Midwife-led continuity models versus other models of care for childbearing women.' *Cochrane Database of Systematic Reviews 4.* Art. No.: CD004667.

Scaer, R.C. (2005) *The Trauma Spectrum: Hidden Wounds and Human Resiliency.* New York: W.W. Norton & Company.

Schiller, R. (2016) 'The women hounded for giving birth outside the system.' *The Guardian,* 22 October. Accessed on 12/12/18 at www.theguardian.com/lifeandstyle/2016/oct/22/hounded-for-giving-birth-outside-the-system.

Schiraldi, G.R. (2009) *The Post-Traumatic Stress Disorder Sourcebook: A Guide to Healing, Recovery, and Growth.* London: McGraw-Hill Education.

Sehhatie, F., Najjarzadeh, M., Zamanzadeh, V. and Seyyedrasooli, A. (2014) 'The effect of midwifery continuing care on childbirth outcomes.' *Iranian Journal of Nursing and Midwifery Research 19*, 3, 233–7.

Simkin, P. (1991) 'Just another day in a woman's life? Women's long-term perceptions of their first birth experience. Part I.' *Birth 18*, 4, 203–10.

Simkin, P. and Klaus, P. (2004) *When Survivors Give Birth: Understanding and Healing the Effects of Early Sexual Abuse on Childbearing Women.* Seattle: Classic Day Publishing.Smith, M. (1998) 'Childbirth in women with a history of sexual abuse (I).' *Practising Midwife 1*, 5, 20–3.

Smith, M. (1998) 'Childbirth in women with a history of sexual abuse.' *Practising Midwife 1*, 5, 20–3.

Soet, J.E., Brack, G.A. and Dilorio, C. (2003) 'Prevalence and predictors of women's experience of psychological trauma during childbirth.' *Birth 30*, 1, 36–46.

Spinelli, M.G. (1997) 'Interpersonal psychotherapy for depressed antepartum women: a pilot study.' *American Journal of Psychiatry 154*, 7, 1028–30.

Spinelli, M.G., Endicott, J., Goetz, R.R. and Segre, L.S. (2016) 'Reanalysis of efficacy of interpersonal psychotherapy for antepartum depression versus parenting education program: initial severity of depression as a predictor of treatment outcome.' *Journal of Clinical Psychiatry 77*, 4, 535–40.

Takehara, K., Noguchi, M., Shimane, T. and Misago, C. (2014) 'A longitudinal study of women's memories of their childbirth experiences at five years postpartum.' *BMC Pregnancy and Childbirth 14*, 221.

Tallman, N. and Hering, C. (1998) 'Child abuse and its effects on birth.' *Midwifery Today with International Midwife 45*, 19–21.

The Telegraph (2015) 'One in three UK female students sexually assaulted or abused on campus.' 14 January. Accessed on 2/8/18 at www.telegraph.co.uk/women/womens-life/11343380/Sexually-assault-1-in-3-UK-female-students-victim-on-campus.html.

Tommys (2019a) 'Pre-eclampsia – information and support.' Accessed on 1/7/19 at www.tommys.org/pregnancy-information/pregnancy-complications/pre-eclampsia-information-and-support.

Tommys (2019b) 'Premature birth – information and support.' Accessed on 1/7/19 at www.tommys.org/pregnancy-information/pregnancy-complications/premature-birth-information-and-support.

Vardo, J.H., Thornburg, L.L. and Glantz, J.C. (2011) 'Maternal and neonatal morbidity among nulliparous women undergoing elective induction of labor.' *Journal of Reproductive Medicine 56*, 1–2, 25–30.

Wood, M., Bartera, C., Stanley, N., Aghtaiea, N. and Larkins, C. (2015) 'Images across Europe: the sending and receiving of sexual images and associations with interpersonal violence in young people's relationships.' *Children and Youth Services Review 59*, 149–60.

Yampolsky, L., Lev-Wiesel, R., Ben-Zion, I.Z. (2010) 'Child sexual abuse: is it a risk factor for pregnancy?' *Journal of Advanced Nursing 66*, 2025–37.

Zepeda Méndez, M., Nijdam, M.J., Ter Heide F.J.J., van der, Aa, N. and Olff, M. (2018) 'A five-day inpatient EMDR treatment programme for PTSD: pilot study.' *European Journal of Psychotraumatology 9*, 1, 1425575.

Zoldbrod, A.P. (2015) 'Sexual issues in treating trauma survivors.' *Current Sexual Health Reports 7*, 1, 3–11.

Zuravin, S., McMillen, C., DePanfilis, D. and Risley-Curtiss, C. (1996) 'The intergenerational cycle of child maltreatment: continuity versus discontinuity.' *Journal of Interpersonal Violence 11*, 3, 315–34.

Index

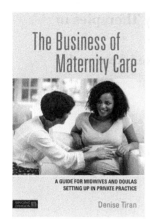

The Business of Maternity Care
A Guide for Midwives and Doulas
Setting Up in Private Practice
Denise Tiran

Paperback: £22.99 / $35.00
ISBN: 978 1 84819 386 4
eISBN: 978 0 85701 385 9
240 pages

This book provides a guide for midwives and doulas who want to establish a maternity-related business offering services such as pregnancy complementary therapies, antenatal classes, lactation support or full doula care. The book is designed to help potential entrepreneurs explore whether this is the right decision for them and provides guidance on the legal, financial and business aspects of setting up in private practice, specifically tailored to maternity care. Advice is given on marketing and pricing and there is debate around the professional and ethical issues for midwives and doulas, including avoiding conflicts of interest and maintaining professional integrity. Case studies of midwives and doulas who have taken the step to set up in private practice are included, and there are various activities to help the reader with their personal plans for their business.

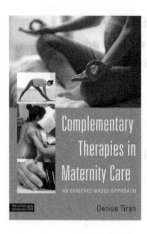

Complementary Therapies in Maternity Care
An Evidence-Based Approach
Denise Tiran

Paperback: £24.99 / $39.95
ISBN: 978 1 84819 328 4
eISBN: 978 0 85701 284 5
352 pages

The complete textbook on complementary therapies in maternity care, this book addresses how midwives and other birth professionals can use or advise on complementary therapies for pregnant, labouring and new mothers. Almost 90% of women may be using complementary therapies during pregnancy and birth, and increasingly midwives and doulas incorporate therapies into their care of women, so it is vital that they and other professionals in the maternity care field are aware of safe and appropriate use based on contemporary evidence. Therapies covered include acupuncture, herbal medicine, homeopathy, aromatherapy, reflexology, yoga, massage and hypnosis.

This complete guide to complementary therapies in pregnancy and childbirth covers safety, effectiveness, evidence, benefits and risks, legal, ethical and professional issues based on accurate and up-to-date research.

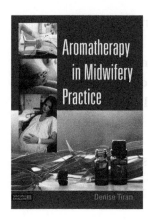

Aromatherapy in Midwifery Practice
Denise Tiran

Paperback: £22.99 / $39.95
ISBN: 978 1 84819 288 1
eISBN: 978 0 85701 235 7
232 pages

Aromatherapy is increasingly incorporated into midwifery practice, particularly in midwife-led units. It is the most commonly used therapy by midwives and birthing practitioners but access to up-to-date safety information is limited. Almost 90% of women may be using complementary therapies during pregnancy and birth and so it is very important that midwives are aware of safe and appropriate use based on contemporary evidence. This book covers safety, effectiveness, evidence, benefits and risks, and legal, ethical and professional issues related to incorporating aromatherapy into maternity care. Useful charts and tables are included for quick reference in clinical practice, making this is the ultimate handbook for using aromatherapy in midwifery practice. The scientific basis behind aromatherapy, including relevant anatomy and physiology, chemistry and pharmacology are covered, as well as a critical appraisal of the contemporary research evidence supporting the use of aromatherapy in maternity care. Essential oil profiles of the oils that can be safely used in pregnancy, birth and postnatally are also included.

Denise Tiran FRCM MSc RM PGCEA is a midwife, lecturer, complementary practitioner and an international authority on maternity complementary medicine. She is Educational Director of Expectancy, which provides academic and professional courses on complementary therapies for midwives, both in the UK and overseas. Denise has recently been honoured with a prestigious Fellowship from the Royal College of Midwives.

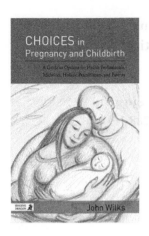

Choices in Pregnancy and Childbirth
A Guide to Options for Health Professionals, Midwives, Holistic Practitioners, and Parents
John Wilks

Paperback: £24.99 / $42.95
ISBN: 978 1 84819 219 5
eISBN: 978 0 85701 167 1
368 pages

Countering increasingly medicalized attitudes towards pregnancy and birth among many healthcare providers, this research-based book discusses the benefits of a more natural approach. It reveals the often-undisclosed effects on a child's long-term development of accepted medical practices, such as induction, C-section, surgical interventions and pain-relief medications. It offers advice on how these practices can be avoided, for example with techniques to encourage optimal foetal positioning, by optimising the birth environment, and through drug-free pain management methods. Ultimately, it enables practitioners to support parents in informed, confident decision-making by giving a balanced account of the complex array of options available throughout pregnancy and birth. With invaluable contributions from midwives, doulas, mothers, and doctors, and tried-and-tested advice on sleep, exercise, diet and therapies, this will a very useful reference for anyone working with women and babies. The information will also be relevant to prospective and new parents.

John Wilks has practiced and taught Craniosacral Therapy and the Bowen Technique for many years and lectures complementary practitioners on pregnancy and childbirth all over the world. He is the author of four books on complementary therapies and developed a specialised Craniosacral training course for midwives which was the first of its kind to be accredited by the Royal College of Midwives. John practices at a multidisciplinary clinic in Dorset, UK.